SHINING THE LIGHT ON PND

THE JOURNEY FROM DARKNESS TO HEALING FROM POST-NATAL DEPRESSION

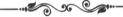

WRITTEN BY

NAMITA MAHANAMA

EDITOR: FELICITY KAY

Shining the Light on PND
Copyright © 2022 by Namita Mahanama

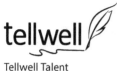

Tellwell Talent
www.tellwell.ca

ISBN
978-0-2288-6296-3 (Hardcover)
978-0-2288-6295-6 (Paperback)
978-0-2288-6297-0 (eBook)

Thank you Felicity for helping me polish
this piece and for making this such a wonderful
process working together. You are amazing!

CONTENTS

DEDICATION

To all of you beautiful mothers navigating your way through this journey of post-natal depression, may we collectively honour your path however difficult, arduous, strenuous and dark it may be right now.

We see you. We feel you. We acknowledge you and what you are going through.

May we forever be here to support, listen and help shine the light on *your* next step forward as we continue to unveil and understand more about this condition as a society.

I promise you beautiful woman, if we hold hands together with unconditional love, compassion, understanding, connection and divine wisdom...that you can venture through this journey with greater ease, lightness, trust and eternal surrender that you *will* heal and you *will* get through this. I promise.

I promise that by using your voice and speaking up for help, that *this* is the first brave step towards your recovery. By acknowledging that you are not feeling your best self, use this bravery to allow you to access all of the tools, resources, support, patience and unconditional love that you deserve, as you embark upon your recovery.

My purpose is to shine the light on post-natal depression so that you and our women in future generations *no longer* have to suffer in silence as I did. It is so that *your* whole world knows how to help you through this journey with the dignity and the support that you deserve.

Keep holding on. You've got this beautiful woman, one day and one breath at a time x

As a dedication to all of you women now and in generations to come, I am donating ten percent of all profits from this book and my children's book *'My Mummy After Our Baby - A Journey Of Hope and Healing'* to the **Gidget Foundation**.

This is a not-for-profit organisation, that is so passionate and dedicated to supporting the emotional well-being of expectant and new mothers. My wish is to generously donate in hope of creating more services and reach to as many beautiful women as possible who deserve to recover from PNDA. It was setup by family and friends of those who lost a beautiful woman nicknamed Gidget to PND and they set this foundation up to help all of the Gidgets out there. I would love nothing more than for them to continue doing their beautiful work.

This is my commitment to paving a path for women enduring this journey to no longer suffer alone and to have access to the best services as you all deserve x

ACKNOWLEDGEMENTS

To my beautiful boys; what can I say that will ever be enough? You breathed a new life into me that I never thought was possible. You shook me to my core and brought me to my knees of who I truly am. Your arrival into the Earth has given me purpose in and of itself, but you have guided me into my dharma and life's purpose to be a vehicle of support for other women experiencing what I did.

You are my *greatest* teachers and I am so thankful with *every* cell in my being that you chose me to be your mother. I will spend the rest of my lifetime showing you how grateful I am for having you in my life and I am so deeply sorry for my disappearance in those first eleven weeks that we had together. I love you with every breath that I take; now and forever more. I would suffer again and again to have you in my world as you have filled my whole entire heart.

To my strong husband Chandi; thank you for holding on and giving me the time and space to heal and recover through this dark and heavy journey. I thank you for trekking through this weathered terrain and for facing each challenge head on with strength and for never giving up. Whilst every day was not easy, nor what one would hope for in their life, I know that you showed up despite feeling defeated, deflated and so profoundly wondering what you did to deserve all of this; though you never said it. I am forever grateful that we continue to show up and heal what we need to when those aspects do arise and face them with an open heart and open communication.

To my amazing parents, beautiful sister Geeta and compassionate brother Yash; thank you for never ever giving up on me and for giving every ounce of your love, dedication, time and parts of yourselves to carry me through this painful path. Your love, guiding light and trust gave me all the strength I needed to carry forth one step at a time. I am grateful in ways that I may never be able to articulate, but feel from the depths of my soul.

To my wonderful 'in-laws' who treated me like their daughter and held my hand in ways I am humbly grateful for. You helped without question, doing all of the parts of life that needed attending to, but I was unable to, and you were there for us when we needed you the most. With silence. With presence. Without judgement. With an open heart, open arms and open mind. Thank you. Though those words may never be sufficient in explaining how I truly feel in my heart.

To all of my Earth angels who helped me along the way, I am eternally grateful. To my two amazing obstetricians that brought my beautiful boys into the world and cared for me even after I delivered and demonstrated true empathy and compassion, thank you. You will remain in my heart forever, as you gave me a family and you gave me my life back by steering me to the help that I needed. I will be eternally grateful to you both.

To my specialists and support team who I met throughout my journey, thank you for never giving up on me and taking the reins when I was completely vulnerable and lost, and steered me towards my recovery at every point throughout this time.

To my Aunty, I will forever *know* that you are my kindred Earth angel the way you helped me in both of my times of distress and despair.

I feel indebted to you for *all* that you did for us and my heart is so grateful to have had you when we needed you the most. I will never truly know how to thank you enough, as any words or actions will never be able to articulate all that I feel.

I am *so* grateful to have had my tribe holding me throughout my healing. I felt supported and *never* alone; which is my wish for every other mother going through this. Find your tribe and lean on them so they can share and lighten the burden on your shoulders and heart as you deserve.

PREFACE

I have been silent for too long. I have a story that now, more than ever before, is so important to share. A story about survival. A story about overcoming darkness in a place and time that is not spoken about enough. A story of two Earth shattering, soul breaking and almost life destroying post-natal depressions. A story that I cannot keep silent any longer.

I release the shame, guilt, embarrassment and taboo or stigma that is attached to suffering from post-natal depression. I wear my war wounds proudly in hope that I can shine the light for those women and families who see no way out of the trenches. I speak out in hope of creating change in a condition that is widely misunderstood, to create opportunities for healing holistically and change the current model where women can get lost in the system, and can lose their lives battling this silent and very isolating dis-ease.

I have two beautiful boys, who are now seven and three as I write this, whom I love with my *entire* heart and soul. They have made me cross into matrescence (think adolescence but from woman into mother) and opened my heart wider to feel things I could never have imagined! They have taught me to be present, to smell the roses, to not sweat the small stuff (and I have learned that it is ALL small stuff!). They have allowed for an internal growth that has shifted so many outdated paradigms, thoughts and mindsets that no longer serve me. For that alone I am *so* eternally grateful for my boys choosing me to be their mother and I promise to love, guide, nurture, honour and protect them in their lives as they so beautifully deserve.

Their arrival did however, bring me to my knees in ways I would never wish upon my worst enemy. Our boys were planned, wanted and craved for with *every* fibre of our being, so what came after each of their births whilst not alone, was certainly soul crushing for all of us; myself, my husband, my children, parents, in-laws and siblings.

Post-natal depression reportedly affects 1 in 7 women in Australia and is the leading cause of maternal death in the first 12 months post-partum. Perinatal mental health, which includes the period of pregnancy, affects 1 in 5 women, which can affect up to 100,000 families each year. This would mean that as of writing this book, based on the number of women alone and assuming that they all had children, (mindfully and sensitively aware that not all women do, would like to or can have children), statistically *1.8 million women* could potentially suffer from PND in Australia. My severity of PND according to my doctor, affects 1 percent of the population and whilst seemingly small, that is still an astronomical number of women, their children, their spouses and parents drowning in the all-encompassing suffering.

It also means that of the almost *300,000* mothers that gave birth in 2018 in Australia (most recent statistic) that almost *42,000* women had PND and *3,000* women had it as severely as I did that year. Knowing the pain and suffering that we endured during our experience, my heart *aches* knowing that so many families have had to or may suffer the pain of this in the future.

Looking at the entire world's population and the number of women there are, and assuming again that they all have children, statistically alone that *could* mean that *532 million women* may suffer from post-natal depression and if 1 percent suffer to the extent that I had it, it would mean that statistically *5.3 million women* could potentially suffer from the effects.

These are NOT small numbers. This is not irrelevant or a passing paragraph to skip through in an antenatal pamphlet when pregnant. This is HUGE.

Yet, why aren't we talking about this? Why do we suffer in silence and feel a *huge* sense of failure? Why do we hide when it is a biochemical cascade that crumbles our whole world, and is of *no* fault of our own just like as if we were to have suffered from any other post-birth complication? Why is there still so much taboo, hiding our wounds and a lack of transparency as to what it is like to live and breathe with day after day?

Life after having a baby isn't always rainbows, butterflies and cute pictures of outfits or 'cookie cutter', 'Instagram-worthy' moments. It can be the harsh reality of wanting to disappear from the world, in a society that expects you to be on top of the moon with love, happiness and joy. This disconnect between the two, creates an even bigger divide, harder expectations to meet and solidifies this stigma that there *is* something wrong with feeling this way when in fact, it is *so* far beyond our control.

There is a genuine misconception held that PND is quite simply the inability to cope with motherhood. Yet, it is due to the biochemical changes in the brain that causes a plethora of symptoms that range from woman to woman, that in fact is what *causes* these feelings. It is often seen as a sign of weakness, however if this is replaced with understanding and empathy, then we create space for the mother to feel comfortable in being open and honest about how she is feeling.

Through the contrast of my illness and wellness, I can fully grasp the fact that PND has a completely different experience around motherhood during that time than without it. Period. My days now are in stark contrast; filled with joy and light compared to my long and heavy days trapped within that darkness.

I want to shine light on the experience; what it can look and feel like, the effects physically, emotionally and on the family unit as a whole. I want you to know that if you are going through it, that you are not alone in how you feel. I also want for those closest to you to help identify if perhaps you do need to reach out for some help, if you are unable to recognise that within yourself. My genuine hope is to inspire and uplift you in the knowing that there *is* light beyond this tunnel and whilst you may feel like there is no way out of the trenches, I promise you *there is*.

I feel that as a pharmacist, I knew all about the medications and the symptoms of PND in 'theory' but being in the thick of it, I did not have the cognitive ability in the deep depression to construct any of my thoughts. There is a stigma around medication for mental health disorders, that it will 'make you a zombie', 'unable to feel and have emotion or opinions'. Yet, medication 100 percent saved my life. Twice.

Never before had I suffered from anxiety or depression, yet, I had severe ideations and without medication I am frightened to think of what my other reality could have been for myself and family.

As a health care professional here in Australia where voicing our own human fallibility is marred with fear of our ability to practise, it is crucial to stand up for all of those suffering in silence, to say that it is OK to reach out and seek support and to not be frightened any longer. How many doctors have taken their own lives, not necessarily to PND but mental health conditions at large; so how many of our health professionals suffer in silence because of fear?

As an Australian-born Indian, deep within our culture is embedded the thought and mindset that conditions related to mental health are signs of weakness and that it is not to be spoken about openly. It gives rise to a 'keeping up with the Kumar's' (pardon the pun!). Not necessarily in a competitive way, but more keeping your silence that anything is 'not OK' and keeping up the charade of a great life, with immense silence of any pain or suffering. It is so easy to speak about our achievements and accomplishments but somehow heavy concepts of any kind are considered 'taboo'. Pretending is apparently easier than speaking the truth and being authentic. No doubt I have seen this to be true in the Chinese, Sri Lankan and South East Asian cultures generally, and to be fair, it is probably present in all cultures across the world! This is why I query the reported statistics, as who truly knows how many families *actually* suffer in silence in the *fear* of being found out.

I also want to acknowledge just how *cruel* this condition is in case you are feeling guilty for feeling the way that you do. It is *so* utterly unbelievably cruel for any condition to completely annihilate your ability to connect and bond with this precious baby, that no doubt you have longed for in your arms for as long as you can remember. Yet, within a blink of an eye, unbeknownst to you, that bond and connection disappears into the ether. How can anyone do that to a mother and the bond with her child? The one she grew in her womb? The one that she is growing? The one that she is raising? If there is a hell here on Earth, if hell does in fact exist, then *this* would be a wonderful picture (amongst others of course) of what it would look like. You have *every* right to feel angry, frustrated, disappointed, 'ripped off' that it happened to you...because I hand on my heart would not wish this upon anybody. I see you and I *completely* understand.

Yet, beyond this layer of frustration, I want to scream from the rooftops that there *is* a way out of how you are feeling. I want to help remind you of *your* why, your anchor into this Earth and to inspire you to make a commitment to yourself that you will take whatever steps that are necessary towards your healing and recovery. Through seeing that healing and recovery *is* possible, my hope is that I can offer you the life support system that you need at a time when you need it the most.

Do not stay back in fear any longer.

Overcoming post-natal depression requires a strength like no other.

I want to start the conversation across the globe of *true* understanding of this condition. People such as your neighbour, friend or work colleague, if they see that your family is suffering and do not have the time, ability or capacity to utilise the resources, that *they* can help navigate you with the arms of solidarity and support. The more people who know about what it looks and feels like by shining the light on PND, then the more they can be there to support you in your recovery and the easier it will be to speak up for help.

As an important note, I want to place a trigger warning potentiality on Part 1 of the book, as it delves deeply into *exactly* how I was thinking and feeling during the depths of my illness. If you are currently experiencing symptoms and feel that reading it will be too confronting or triggering, then please skip straight to chapter 3 of Part 1 or straight to Part 2 where you can simply access the reflections, learnings and tools that I have to share, rather than feeling worse than you may already feel by reading the rawness of my experiences.

The rawness is being shared only in hope that if you are sitting on the fence undecided if you have PND, that this will make it crystal clear as to what it can look and feel like, so that you do not delay walking towards your recovery. It also allows an opportunity for family members to recognise that if the mother is unable to 'reach out' or 'speak out', that they can 'reach in' and help guide her towards the help that is required. It is to cover all bases, so that *all* support people know what it can look and feel like to have post-natal depression, and to map out some very clear action steps to take.

It will fill my heart with *so* much gratitude that despite those darkest times, the pain that my family went through was not in vain and that something good has come out of it, if it helps carry *you* over to the side of healing and recovery.

HOW SHOULD I READ THIS BOOK?

+ If you are able to concentrate, focus and have the energy to do so, then certainly read it from start to finish; which begins with my experiential story then moves onto more of a factual resource

+ Otherwise, skip to exactly the parts that you feel may benefit you the most. I know that in the depths of sleep deprivation and depression; or caring for someone with PND, reading a long book in its entirety may not be very practical...so go exactly to the parts that are most helpful to you in the moment and stage that you are in

+ This is designed to be a **survival guide** where you can turn and go to whatever is relevant to you at the time directly. Go to what resonates and what will help you perfectly in that moment

+ Go to Chapter 11 of Part 2 of the book for a **'Summary of all tools as a quick reference guide'** which are the tools in summation without all of the 'fluff' writing

+ I have written a summary list of my reflections, mindsets and tools for the mother before the full explanation of each one, if you want to skip to a particular one instead of reading it in its entirety

+ There may be repeated information in various sections for completeness and wholeness sake for those that are flipping to different sections. This has been done to ensure that you understand the concept in full no matter how you decide to utilise this resource

+ Go to the Q and A section in Chapter 1 of Part 2 if that style resonates with you, as it spells out exactly the ins and outs of PND

+ As mentioned earlier, my story in Part 1 may be *triggering* for some, so I encourage you to skip past it if it brings up any uninvited feelings... If triggering, you can read Chapter 3 only of Part 1 or skip straight to Part 2 of the book for the pearls of wisdom that I collected from the experience

+ The glossary has the full meaning for the words in Sanskrit used throughout, as well as the abbreviations used. PND (post-natal depression) and PNDA (perinatal anxiety and depression; meaning the period throughout pregnancy and/or post-partum) have been used interchangeably but have one and the same meaning here

PART 1

MY STORY

When I first began reflecting through my journey, I recounted every aspect of my life all the way from childhood to present day as a way to reflect and understand my entire journey and possibly why I ended up here. This process was extremely cathartic and allowed for me to come to my understandings about my learnings, mindsets and patterns.

Sharing my feelings during pregnancy and my post-natal depression hopefully will allow you to identify similarities with how you are feeling. My hope is that by being raw and honest in how I felt at the time, it will allow you to connect with the fact that you are *not alone* in what you are going through and that how you are feeling *is* the condition. I also want to share the vast experience of life and love that I have been able to embrace upon my recovery, to enable you to see that reaching out for help *is* the first brave step and that what lies past this road is so abundantly bountiful and that *you can* experience this too.

My boys are my whole world. I live and breathe for them. I savour every sacred moment with them because I know what that disconnection felt like, so I do not take for granted my cognition and ability to think and feel as I do now. Part of me still feels awful that I denied these pure and innocent souls their mother's love and pure connection in those early 11-weeks. They didn't deserve that nor have any idea what had happened to their mother that they chose to come through.

I have had to make peace and forgive myself for having post-natal depression and for understanding that it occurred through no fault of my own. I now stand in my power in knowing that I rose up to heal and recover from it and have become completely present with them and am able to give them the very best of me each and every day. This may be as a form of redemption, but also making sure that I give them the best of me now that I am in health and wellness as they *absolutely* deserve.

You deserve to feel so connected to the whole of life itself; to your children, partner, family and each and every breath that you take. You *deserve* to *feel* joy, clarity of mind, energy, optimum vitality and *all* of this is available to you if you can identify and be honest with *exactly* how you are feeling and can identify that it is contrasting to your true self. Then allow either yourself to take that first step, or allow those closest to you to reach out their hand and to carry you over to the side of recovery and healing.

We are humans and it is OK to be fallible, it truly is. It is not a sign of weakness in saying that you do not feel like yourself and it *is* in the rising up where the real sweetness lies. The rising up, stepping forward and allowing for the healing to occur in whatever ways that *you* need, requires a strength like no other. The strength that you will carry forth into your days moving forward from this will be *so* empowering to your children and other women in your world.

Treat this chapter in your life with the same kindness and compassion that you would if you had fallen over and broken your leg. If this happened, then without judgement or any feelings attached, you would go to the hospital, have your leg placed in a cast, take any medication that was prescribed for the pain and rest. You would happily accept help from family and friends to prepare meals, collect older children and do small errands for you. You would most likely then go to a physiotherapist and learn the exercises that you need to strengthen the joint and muscles around it, until the area has healed and you can confidently place weight on your leg.

Recovering from post-natal depression is no different, except that your pain does not have an outward symbol of trauma in the same way as it does for a broken leg. Whilst this may not allow others to see your pain, this does *not* minimise your condition. At all. You require rest, rejuvenation and nourishment to your body after giving birth, whilst exploring the treatment options available for your specific symptoms and biochemical imbalance that presents. In time, allowing yourself to heal and restore your biochemistry; which is akin to having a cast on the broken bone with pain relief, and doing Cognitive Behavioural Therapy (CBT) or IPT (Interpersonal Therapy); which is akin to physiotherapy, these will allow you to confidently step forward in your life with the balance and coping tools or strategies that you require.

Remove any judgement, remove the stigma and shame that you may attach about feeling the way that you do and *allow* yourself the opportunity to return back into your light. Staying stuck where you are and feeling less than wonderful is not the best way to live life. Imagine the feelings of joy and pleasure in your life again where now there may only be darkness, sadness and an inability to function at your capacity.

Whilst parenthood will *always* have challenging moments, days and periods which can feel extremely exhausting, isolating, lonely and the compelling need to be seen, held and supported from your tribe...for example home schooling during Covid lockdown with two or three children at home, it is normal and natural to feel the frustration and stress. We are humans at the end of the day and our children *do* test the patience of anyone especially with being in confined spaces, financial stress, when they are fighting or there is constant noise and mess...not to mention throwing in illness to an already exhausting day! It is no wonder that it takes a village to raise a child. However, I still do feel that this is manageable when your brain biochemistry is *balanced*. One can draw on the inner resilience to get through the chaos that is, but with imbalanced biochemistry with PND it can be enough to make you feel like you cannot go on.

I would say that being in the depths of post-natal depression with my heart and brain centre obsolete; that I would choose feeling 1000 days of normal parenting realities than even one more hour of how I felt during that time. Hands down.

I would also say that treatment may not be black and white as everyone's symptoms and presentations may be different. Yet, the one thing that stands in the way of you feeling your best self or remaining in how you feel right now, is first identifying then accepting that you are feeling unwell. This will then allow you to take that *first step* into speaking up and seeking help from your GP, obstetrician, midwife or child health nurse and being completely honest about how you are feeling.

Once you have made this brave step then what will unfold has the potential to be so magical and transformative to you as a person. The person that I am today is a stronger, more aligned, more connected and truly present version of the person I was before I endured all of this. Sometimes through hitting rock bottom we can rise up into who we always had the potential to become, and we drop the 'small stuff' and just savour the magic that is all around us.

This is all available to you too x

CHAPTER 1

BABY ARI

When we as a couple felt ready to embark upon the journey of parenthood, I fell pregnant with Ari quite easily on the second month of trying. We felt very grateful and blessed as to the ease of this part of the process as we felt so ready and were longing to have a baby. We know that a lot of people do have very long and difficult paths to conceive, so we were grateful for the ease in this part of our journey.

I knew intuitively that we were having a little boy, as he felt very masculine in essence and even now as a 7-year old, he is my masculine spirit. My pregnancy was very seamless and ticked along without any real concerns or troubles. I felt extremely connected to him and I was *so* excited to meet him and have him in our lives.

As a first-time pregnant woman and Mum-to-be, I read a lot about the growth and stages of development of him in utero but did not read a lot about optimal foetal positioning, as I felt that having a natural delivery would be just something that my body would organically go through.

We were living in Cairns for business whilst our home and family were all in Sydney, so we were isolated away from our 'tribe' during this time. We felt that our parents had raised us both without extended family so it was something that whilst being challenging, that we'd be able to get through.

I had stopped working as a full-time pharmacist at 6 months into my pregnancy as I found standing 9-10 hours a day quite challenging with fluid retention and the amount of weight that I had gained. I had thrown caution to the wind and was literally eating for two... or three...or four, overindulging and ended up gaining a whopping 33kg! I hadn't realised the weight creeping up on me and decided to weigh myself the day I went into labour and was *mortified*; and now, even more mortified that I am writing this number down!

We excitedly prepared for his arrival with a beautiful nursery, pram and all the gadgets that new parents proudly gather. We went to our antenatal classes and never thought about post-natal depression aside from a slide in our class and possibly a Beyond Blue pamphlet that we received in our 'goodie bag'. I thought I had seen depression in so many patients and knew the symptoms in 'theory' that I would be able to identify it in myself if it happened, so parked it on the shelf as something I didn't want to place too much attention on.

HOSPITAL

I went into labour three days before his estimated due date with my waters breaking and proceeded to the hospital waiting for it to progress. I then had the induction drip and gel to allow progress on a labour that was becoming more and more painful and not progressing *at all*. As it turned out after a 30-hour exhausting, painful labour, Ari was not in the right position and had become completely lodged inside my pelvis which resulted in an emergency caesarean.

I remember feeling extremely defeated at this point as if my body had let me down and that if a 'natural delivery' was so natural, effortless, and what our bodies were born to do, then mine was a complete failure. I felt like I hadn't prepared myself for a C-section and the recovery that it would entail, not being able to drive and I was completely unsure how I would look after a baby with a huge cut in my stomach and womb. This was catastrophic and very dramatic thinking, given that so many women have a caesarean and many more complex medical conditions! However, similar to the post-natal depression leaflet and slide, I skipped past the C-section part thinking that it wouldn't be relevant to me, perhaps more as a naïve ideology of where attention goes, energy flows so I didn't want to harp too much on it as I assumed I would have a natural delivery.

I was also so exhausted and still in pain, so equally there was so much relief that soon I would see our little boy, hold him in my arms and all of this would be a distant memory and I could move forward with having a rest and just enjoy my beautiful baby. I also felt relief by this point, as it was still Thursday 12th and I desperately wanted to avoid him being born on Friday 13th. My controlling nature thought that I could govern his birth-day as if I were some master orchestrator of his journey, path and life...I can only giggle now about the absurdity of this!

At around 11.45pm my amazing obstetrician said 'Get ready to say Happy Birthday'. It then took a turn in becoming slightly eventful, as he was severely wedged within my pelvis. My obstetrician required a lot of force and energy using forceps, the table was shaking from her using all of her muscle and grit and I remember trembling. It could have been the combination of adrenaline coupled with the epidural, but the anaesthetist was holding my arm as it was trembling and shaking so much. Eventually 19 minutes later from all of this forceful tugging and pulling him out, Ari was born at 12.04am on Friday 13th. The relief was immense and the joy and love we felt was in abundance. Yet, I now continue to giggle thinking that those four minutes past midnight showed me that I *cannot* nor can I *ever* control him and what his destiny or journey is. One of my first lessons in relinquishing control during this journey of motherhood.

Our first few days in the hospital were initially full of relief, joy, happiness, excitement, yet also fatigue, given the long thirty hours of labour. The endorphins and oxytocin filled me with happiness and connection and we were in a beautiful love bubble.

However, from the outset I had enormous trouble with breastfeeding Ari, having issues with attachment and milk supply. Ari would scream upon latching and would cry so much that his whole face and body would turn bright red. I called the midwives at each feed to help me latch and make sure I was attaching him correctly, knowing that eventually I would need to be able to do this alone, so I had to capitalise on the beautiful help of the nurses. Every second feed brought upon a new nurse with different advice as to how to attach and slowly as the fatigue wore in, I slowly started to dread each feed time knowing that it would be met with crying and the pain was excruciating.

From the morning of day 4, I started to feel my anxiety set in with a feeling of pins and needles initially on my chest and neck, which palpably felt like a heaviness on my chest. Up until this point I had never suffered from anxiety but I could physically feel the effects within my body, so I knew that something was not quite right. Though, I did not place two and two together at this early stage.

My mouth felt constantly dry and when I spoke I felt extremely aware of this feeling. My mind started racing from one thought to the next and I could not fall asleep even if Ari was sleeping. I felt my mind starting to become very 'wired' and I was unable to relax and just 'be'. When he was sleeping, I would be anxious and dreading the next feed and often would hand express so I had enough milk ready to use when he woke up again. I hoped that having milk ready would stop him escalating to the bright red screaming that I was met with every 2 hours. I felt like I was 'on' all the time despite knowing that my body desperately needed sleep and yet, I could not switch off.

The feeds then progressed to me hand expressing and cup feeding, though my supply was not extensive. Then we moved onto syringe feeding which was better, as the cup was causing him to regurgitate and spit it back up as it was too fast. Then we progressed to line feeding...if you are feeling overwhelmed with your breastfeeding journey, you are not alone in this crazy choreography, so do not despair!

There was talk from the nurses that giving the bottle and dummy can cause confusion with the latch and he may have trouble going back and forth. We did use a dummy to settle him because he was crying and unsettled so much and truly, the poor bubba was clearly just hungry!

With each passing moment, my anxiety was getting stronger and I had not slept *at all*, not even a minute or a second of sleep. I started to dread every noise that Ari made as I felt like I could not help him. I couldn't feed him, though I breastfed with an audience of very experienced nurses at each and every feed. I felt so overwhelmed and out of my depth. Did I feel this way from my anxiety or did feeling this way cause my anxiety? Or was it the direct impact that my change in pregnancy hormones to breastfeeding hormones was causing on my biochemistry?

From my reflection I was so determined to breastfeed my baby at whatever cost because I had been trained and told that 'breast is best', and I put this pressure on myself that I had to breast feed him. I felt that my body had failed me giving birth to him naturally, that at least I couldn't fail in being able to feed him in this most natural and primal base connection way. I am a woman and now a mother so I *should* be able to do this, right? Yet, this pressure that I put on myself made me feel worse and worse about myself every time I fed him. The sleep deprivation coupled with my anxiety at each feed propelled me further into the feelings of anxiety, which became a vicious cycle that ultimately affected my milk supply!

On the day before we went home, I tried latching him for so long with a nurse who began sweating profusely from the whole thing. I was becoming even more anxious with shallower breaths, felt shaky with Ari screaming his head off, and all three of us were becoming unravelled, that she eventually suggested giving him formula. She explained that he was just so hungry and he would continue to have negative associations with the breast if we continued.

I felt tremendous guilt. I felt like a huge failure. I felt like the worst mother in the world that was denying her child of the nutrition that he deserved. I felt so resentful of my body for not performing the way nature had intended and all of these feelings ran through my head, instead of sleeping like my body so desperately needed... again very dramatic and catastrophic thinking.

So we fed Ari formula and thankfully he took it well and actually never had any issues with it throughout his entire time. I continued to express in hope that he would latch and I could feed, or if not at least express and bottle feed him because I wanted to do the best for him. I felt like the nursing staff felt a sense of relief at this point since we had tried everything at every single feed, and we were just not making any head way.

The next morning on day 5, when my milk officially came in, I had literally 'gone', 'disappeared' and 'vanished' overnight. It felt like I had entered into this heavy black-zipped cloak and my smile had disappeared and the essence of me had walked out the door. I was unable to have a proper conversation, my mind was feeling like a cloudy, spaced-out fog and it felt like there was a black cloud engulfing my entire being. I was filled with so much dread that I was being sent home and I had no idea what to do.

My blood pressure was high for the first time in my life, but the nurse sensed that I may feel better once we were home as she knew the tiring time that we had at the hospital. We were discharged and Chandi said he was hopeful that being at home would 'reset' us and that I would be able to sleep, eat and feel myself again. I remember being in the car on the drive home, telling myself to 'snap out of it' and 'pull it together' and rationalise that I was coming home with a beautiful healthy baby and that I had absolutely *no reason* to feel this way. I tried to imagine that nothing had gone wrong and I needed to get myself together and feel happy to be going home. I would have moments of feeling optimistic but the general mood and tone were of absolute dread, wanting to bury my head under the blanket and just forget this whole ordeal had ever happened! I felt pasty, exhausted beyond belief and the thought of still having to look after Ari and feed him felt so overwhelming for me.

HOME

Thankfully Chandi's Mum had come from Sydney before Ari was born and was there to help us for the first two weeks until my parents came up from Sydney also. She helped us so much with the cooking, cleaning and taking Ruphus our dog for walks, that we would have been in a world of pain had we not had any help during these early stages. I am *so* grateful that she was our lifeline during this time and helped without question in every way that she could.

The way I felt steadily became worse as the hours went by. My anxiety was now present 24/7, with it feeling like hot knives cutting my chest and neck and would radiate going down my arms. I still could not sleep, even for 5 minutes despite trying time...and time... and time again. I know Chandi thought that if I *just* slept I would feel better but I literally could *not* go to sleep. I was *so* wired and yet, I felt like a zombie too where I could not construct any sentences or could not make *any* decisions.

11

I could not smile and any aspect of pleasure, joy or happiness was absolutely impossible.

I would look into space and either mindlessly think or tell whoever was near me things like, I 'should have done' or 'should not have done' this, that or the other and blamed myself for feeling this way.

I would continuously go off on a tangent loop of regret about having a baby; 'what have I done? I shouldn't have had a baby...I'm stuck with this baby for the rest of my life that I don't know how to take care of'.

I felt so trapped in this new role and saw no respite, no hope or light at the end of the tunnel.

I thought I would never sleep again, and I was to the bone exhausted.

I could not eat a bite of food.

I could not sleep even for a minute. Not even a second. Tossing and turning with one incessant thought to the next.

I went from a woman who wanted a baby with *every* cell in her being, to one who was saying such hurtful and irrational things. This was the *biggest* indicator of post-natal depression above all of the other physical symptoms of anxiety and low mood. We did however, just hold on thinking that it would get better in time, and still at this point did not think it was anything more sinister than a case of the Baby Blues...or sleep deprivation coupled with a long labour and hormone changes.

The next few days I fell further and further into the *deepest* depression which was sinking me into even more incognisant thoughts. I could not choose clothes to wear and would stand in front of my cupboard for an hour (not exaggerating). I could not make decisions on what I felt like eating together with zero appetite, so ended up not eating at all. I would get lost with time completely and rather than rest when I could, I would try to express milk or Google whatever crazy thoughts that came into my head. My anxiety was worsening and it physically hurt my chest and neck, *especially* when I was 'trying' to sleep. It was as if the silence made my symptoms undeniably palpable.

We spoke to my beautiful midwife Jillian at my obstetrician's practice, who was so incredibly supportive and understanding. My obstetrician prescribed some sleeping medication to hopefully allow me to get to sleep, as we all felt that the insomnia was the limiting factor into allowing me to feel better.

Unfortunately, they did not work at all and I continued to be 'wired' and my thoughts continued to run wild.

My Mother-in-law thought that it would be helpful for her to sleep with Ari in his nursery instead of next to me in our room, hoping that allowing me to sleep undisturbed even for a short while would help me feel better. Yet, I still could not sleep and the guilt that riddled me that my baby was not next to me, added to my feelings of shame and worsened how I was feeling. It still amazes me even today, the depth of feelings that arise when biochemistry is off balance, and it has the ability to make us feel worse and worse no matter what solution is presented. I constantly just wanted to hide under a blanket and disappear from all of this ridiculousness.

I decided to stop expressing after coming to the realisation that my milk supply was still remarkably low and that my sleep deprivation was not helping my supply. I also felt that perhaps the breastfeeding hormones could be what was causing me to feel this way after a conversation with the child health nurse that eluded to this possibility. Stopping this unsuccessful and unnecessary step felt like the right thing to do. Whilst I felt guilty for not giving Ari the best possible nutrition, I *had* to change something as the current recipe of what I was doing was not working for me.

Thankfully I didn't get mastitis or blocked milk ducts from stopping expressing or feeding immediately. I used cabbage leaves to help with the swelling and heat that ensued but I was slightly optimistic that this piece of the puzzle may return me back to feeling myself again. I inherently knew that I was not myself but *even* at that point I did not think anything about having post-natal depression. Denial perhaps. Not having the ability to think clearly, blurred my once rational and sensible thought processes.

After a week or so being at home, our business partner and his fiancée, now wife, came to our place. I stood standing at the cupboard again for well over an hour not moving and completely unable to decide what clothes to wear or how to get ready. Normally I am a bright, bubbly person full of conversation, wit and humour, yet I simply sat on the couch like a zombie. I could not smile, participate in any conversation and just not feeling happy *at all*. Where normally I refuel and re-energise from talking with friends, I was a vessel of emptiness.

My Mother-in-law was chatting away and I remember feeling like my loop was the only thing I could think of 'what have I done having a baby, I will never have fun again' and wishing I could just curl up and disappear. They left early as they obviously could see that I was not myself and associated this with needing to recover after my C-section.

My negative loop of regret intensified and grew the more I spoke about it. I would chew everyone's ear off who would listen. I lived in the 'should have, could have, I wish I did this' mode and the more I spoke and thought it, the more it strengthened and grabbed hold of me. I would say that 'someone should have warned me about all of this' and that 'I should have practised with other kids before thinking

I could do this myself'. I used to say silly things like 'I should have put an alarm on every 40 minutes when sleeping and see if I could handle it' and that 'everyone would be better off without me'.

I was spiralling out of control with each hour that passed.

My parents, brother and sister were growing more worried about me from Sydney because I wouldn't answer their calls *at all* or respond to any of their messages. I felt too overwhelmed to answer their calls. How could I possibly explain all that I was feeling without admitting to my awful loop, and I was *so* embarrassed by my behaviour and how I was feeling. I couldn't genuinely write a sentence in a message without it taking 40 minutes so I disappeared completely from my friends, social media and just couldn't reply to anyone at all. With the switch off in my brain, so too did I switch off from the world. If you do ever notice yourself, friends or family who are normally very responsive suddenly disappearing from contact, then do speak up or reach out. It is often a sign of isolating or withdrawing themselves, from being overwhelmed or having anxiety and depression.

Yet, after realising just how worried I was making them, I did answer my parents and siblings calls and just ended up blurting out whatever it was that I was thinking and feeling. Once I started I could not stop. I would then speak with them multiple times throughout the day and it eventually got to a point where I couldn't construct sentences unless it was about my loop. Whilst draining and frustrating for everyone involved, upon reflection I realise that this *was* my strength in coming out of this by week 11, in that I was so articulate in explaining my thought processes, my loop, my sticky and muddy feelings that there was nothing left to anyone's imagination, other than undeniably knowing exactly how I was feeling. This would have been different if perhaps like other conversation points, I was just silent. No one would know what I was thinking or feeling and I could potentially have been stuck in this mud for much longer. I commend myself on this ability to speak up and articulating my thoughts even in the depths of this despair, and I do genuinely believe it is what allowed me to show others how much help I did in fact need.

My parents were booked to come at the two-week mark but my beautiful sister was so worried about me that she dropped *everything* and flew up after around a week. She stayed one night as she was flying out the next day on an overseas trip, but desperately wanted to see what was going on and how I was doing. It was a short sharp session that I am *so grateful* for, as she dropped her entire life with her three young children, especially appreciating the logistics involved with travel now with my own two boys, to come and check in on me. She saw that I was not in any harm's way and like everyone else thought that once I slept, I would be on the road to recovery and continued to be available for me through messages and calls 24/7.

My Dad in those early few weeks I remember was the one that explicitly said that maybe I had post-natal depression. However, no one truly knew enough about what was happening to unequivocally say what it was that I was experiencing. Actually it was my beautiful Dad who gave me the strength and courage to hold on the second time around also, and encouraged me that *when* I get through this (he never had any doubt that I wouldn't) as to how many women I would be able to help through this same experience. His words at the time gave me more of my 'why' to keep holding on and his loving guidance here gave me the strength I needed to pull through day after day knowing that I had to do this for him, myself, my boys and all future women. His support and guiding light will stay with me forever and always.

My beautiful Mum also when I told her upon my recovery that I wanted to set out to help as many women as I could, encouraged me with so much love and kindness. She said that there would be so many women suffering and how much they need this, and whilst it may be hard for the first person to stand up, that it would be so helpful. I can cry just thinking of her loving support in this and everything else this beautiful woman and man have given to me x

My sister and sister-in-law both had several children between them but never experienced this, so there was an element of not knowing exactly what it was that was happening to me. Was it my hormones? Was it my reaction to stress? Was it simply the sleep deprivation causing this? No one knew.

At this point, I can see that I had a lot of red flags and my husband, parents and siblings around me knowing that something wasn't quite right, became the life support system that I needed. They were my outlet and my branch that I clung onto when I felt like I was drowning. Speaking with them every hour sometimes day after day, allowed me to hold faith and strength that I was *not alone* in this. I went from not answering their calls to contacting them *all* the time or speaking to Chandi almost as a diary or outlet from my head. I would articulate every thought I was having, despite it not being things I am proud of saying now. Yet, they listened without judgement. With an open heart, open arms and open ears.

Their unconditional love, guidance and support is what got me through one hour at a time. Sometimes even one moment at a time. Their constant checking-in on me and being the shoulder to lean on was *exactly* what I needed. If I was left to navigate the thoughts in my head alone and not have the ability to talk it through, then I don't know how or even *if* I would have held on. I truly believe that the incessant thoughts, the anxiety, the inability to function and being completely ravaged by these disconnected feelings, would have taken over my entire being and I can only shudder at the thought of the other possible outcome of this. As time wore on, my thoughts became more serious in ideation so I know that without speaking about it to my loved ones, that they could have heightened or actualised.

I felt so bad that I was burdening them all with how I was feeling, being the weight on everyone's shoulders at a time that 'should' be filled with so much joy and happiness and dragging them down with my claws. The same claws that had *their* hold on *me* and my mind, body and soul. They all had their own lives to get through themselves and yet, I absolutely ravaged each of them with pouring my heart and soul onto them. How they managed to go to work, cook dinner/look after their own children, look after their own life and health, as well being available for me 24/7 is a testament to the love and support that I was surrounded by. They were all there for me without question, whether it was my husband and family staying with me or those in Sydney.

I owe them *all* my life. Each and every one of them.

Just after we had approached the 2-week mark Chandi explained that I should call Beyond Blue (an organisation that specialises in mental health support) to speak to someone and see what advice they had. He only had 3-weeks of paternity leave, so time was ticking and I was only getting worse and not living this loved up, baby-infused joyous newborn phase that we expected for us. Rather than sleepless nights from Ari, it was me who was not sleeping and keeping him up from the worry about my health, well-being and safety.

I hesitantly agreed to call Beyond Blue and I remember sitting in the nursery on the chair crippled with anxiety and the inability to feel like I had the strength to call them and start this conversation.

What would I say?

How would they respond?

Will they contact authorities and flag me?

How can anyone fix any of this and get me out of this mess? I genuinely thought that the help I needed, no one could give to me.

I did end up calling them with my heart pounding, mind racing, with a dry mouth, sweating, shaking and feeling like the hot knives were *cutting* into my chest and neck. I explained to the lady at the other end of the phone how I was feeling and it certainly was nice to speak to someone impartial and I did not feel judged *at all*. She was very sweet, gentle and empathetic on the phone. She listened without rushing me and then suggested that I call PANDA (Perinatal Anxiety and Depression Australia), as they are a specialised service for post-natal depression. I had to gather enough strength again to get the courage to call them, as that phone call took all of my energy in and of itself.

I did reluctantly call them, again crippled with fear, anxiety, a racing heart and shaky voice. They suggested that I see my GP and let them know how I was feeling. At this time of not being able to function, the concept of having to make an appointment, leave the house, get dressed with or without the baby seemed like the most mammoth and ridiculous task! I was exhausted from just making these two phone calls let alone trying to book an appointment with a GP, that I had never needed before so didn't have...

So to the doctor I did not go or take any action. I truly in my heart believed that it would just get better on its own and surely what could anyone help me with when it was wishing I didn't have a baby that was the problem? This was my *actual* thought process, and now with health reinstated it sounds so horrendous that I thought any of these things. This beautiful baby *was* wanted, planned for and *so* welcome throughout my whole pregnancy that a thought like that of wishing I never had him, is not a thought that a well mind would think. This thought *alone* would be the sign that I needed help and needed help fast. Whilst I continued with the sleeping tablets that my OB had prescribed, they were not working and the spiral continued.

A child health nurse came to our home twice and I was absolutely petrified and scared that she would know that something was wrong with me and send me into an institution or take my baby away from me. Whilst in theory I knew she was there to help me, it felt so clinical, litigious and I felt like it was very much a 'government watching' approach that made me too fearful to be honest with her. She gave me the EPDS questionnaire (the *Edinburgh Postnatal Depression Scale,* which can be accessed online and is a screening tool for health professionals to gauge how you are feeling after having a baby). I thought if I actually answer the truth I would score so high and that fear crippled me to my core. So I held back. Twice.

The nurse offered for me to join in the mothers' group and I did explain how out of depth I felt and how I didn't feel comfortable joining when all the other mums would know what to do and it's just me who was finding this all too hard. She did reassure me that I wasn't the only one who felt that way and that I should join in. Yet, the thought of being around a group of strangers when I literally couldn't hold a conversation, or took over 45 minutes to make Ari's bottle; was just too much. I felt like a deer in headlights and as dull as a door knob, that the prospect of socialising was *impossible.*

My thoughts continued getting very dark, filled with severe ideations where I would vividly imagine myself escaping from all of this reality.

I felt helpless.

Utterly exhausted.

Unbelievably stuck in mud that I felt like I was being drowned in thick quick sand and drowning in water all at the same time.

I could not possibly imagine what anyone could do or say to make me feel better or to change any of it. I truly saw no light at the end of the tunnel, any future ahead or any glimpses of hope for me.

Yet, even in the midst of all of these horrendously dark thoughts, not once did I realise that it *was* the disease of post-natal depression that was causing *all* of these thoughts. I believed that my regret and disconnection were *so unbelievably* real and tried to convince all those around me that I had made the biggest mistake. Yet, it was the biochemistry that ensued from having my baby which is *what* was wreaking havoc on my body, mind and soul.

I didn't realise even for a second that by taking action and seeking treatment that I could *actually stop* all of this. Every single minute of suffering could stop.

The feeling like I couldn't breathe.

The feeling like I could not eat a morsel of food with zero appetite.

The inability to sleep even a wink. No matter how hard I tried.

The feeling of having a mountain of knives sitting on my chest, every second of every day.

The feeling of my brain being in a thick muddy fog.

The feeling like I was suffocating and drowning all at the same time.

The feeling of such disconnection from this gorgeous, divine and beautiful baby that was the picture of perfection; my dream baby in my arms.

No joy. No heart. No emotion. No connection to *anything*.

The essence of me had vanished.

Fear is what kept me immobilised. Fear is what kept me trapped in this horrible reality.

I wouldn't sleep at all with my thoughts wandering off to negative places, and then I would see the morning roll in and I would bury my head further underneath the blanket just *wishing* I could disappear. Ari would cry and I would just cringe inside like a pit in my stomach or pretend that I didn't hear him. He slept for the first time through the night at 6 weeks, though not a regular feature, but I couldn't even muster any happiness or relief over this amazing feat, as I was too bogged down in my thoughts.

Bogged down in my darkness. Bogged down in thinking that this was going to be my reality. Forever.

I blamed myself for causing this self-inflicted pain and felt like no one could get me out of this horror.

I felt ripped off by my body. I felt resentful to others for not feeling this way. Resentful for nobody warning me that this was possible.

I felt so alone because no one I knew had ever experienced this and I felt like of all the things to be unique for, this would have to be the worst thing of all.

WHAT DID LIFE CONTINUE TO LOOK LIKE AS TIME WENT ON?

I still could not sleep at all. Chandi would stay up all night and look after Ari when he woke up, then would go to work leaving at 7am and coming home at 6.30pm. Thankfully my parents were there after my Mother-in-law went back to Sydney. My Dad stayed for two weeks and then had to go back to work, but my Mum stayed for another three weeks after that to be with me.

During our days together they tried to talk to me about non-loop things, go for walks to change the scenery, cheer me up by watching funny videos or feel-good movies. However, I could not focus on any movies or any T.V shows as my mind would just wander off on my loop. I couldn't find the joy or funny side to *anything* and I became very cynical in seeing people live their lives normally.

When Chandi was super tired, my Mum would help me with Ari throughout the night. She did all of our cooking, our washing, cleaning and looking after Ari when Chandi wasn't there. I did the basics with Ari but the connection wasn't there, and my mind was so foggy that I would get lost in space for hours at a time, just staring blankly into the ether. Thank goodness that they were there to support me otherwise it is a scary prospect as to what could have happened when someone is so severely affected as I was. They were my saviours and kept Ari and me alive.

I owe them my life without a shadow of a doubt.

I would get lost in the Google vortex and research how to get my baby to sleep, even though I wasn't sleeping myself and he slept better than me! I started to read 'Save our Sleep' by Tizzie Hall as I was so adamant that I had to follow this routine for him to sleep, but could obviously hardly focus on the book. I would then get cranky at my Mum or Chandi when they weren't following it or holding him for too long, as I thought when everyone goes back that I would be stuck holding him forever without any help. Catastrophic thinking. They would tell me to throw the book out, that each baby is different and that it was making me feel worse.

I would Google everything and the over-abundance of information, people's opinions on forums and unqualified people giving so much advice, all added to my anxiety and depression tremendously. I would stay in my room and 'try' unsuccessfully to sleep day after day. I hardly changed out of my pyjamas because what was the point and I couldn't get ready anyhow.

Complete loss of any care taken for my aesthetics. Motivation zero. Care factor double zero.

Upon reflection I was an *absolute* mess. How was everyone so patient with me?

I remember this one day before my parents arrived, I went into the kitchen to make Ari's milk, and I stood in the kitchen looking at the oven clock. I walked to the steriliser and just stood there not doing anything, just walking from one place to the other. When I looked at the oven again, a *whole hour* had passed by and I had not done a thing. I literally could not think or function in even very simplistic tasks.

Physical ailments are obvious. Mental ailments especially at a complicated time after birth, where we can justify hormones or sleep deprivation as logical explanations, make it harder to understand or even see sometimes. Not in my case though, as it was clearly evident for all those around me, not necessarily for myself being the actual patient and in the thick of it.

Somehow with the support of our amazing family through all of this darkness, the frustrations and tensions about me incessantly talking about this loop and clearly not making any progress, we got through the first few weeks.

My obstetrician brought forward my 6-week appointment given the state that I was in. I remember being riddled with anxiety and not wanting to go and yet, when I saw my beautiful midwife Jillian, I just burst into tears. I cried and cried and cried. She had seen me throughout my whole pregnancy and this was something she had never seen from me, and knew undoubtedly that I was now in the right place. I said that I was so embarrassed to see my obstetrician because I had a healthy baby and had *no reason* to feel or be acting this way.

Thankfully when I saw my OB, she was incredibly understanding, empathetic, calm, kind and was just present and supportive. She didn't try to minimise my feelings or experience and simply went into solution mode. It was what we needed to create action, as there was complete awareness that something had to change in order for me to recover back into my vibrant and bubbly self.

She immediately gave me a referral to see a psychiatrist and thankfully being in private healthcare, I did not have to wait long. I was able to see her within a few days which I am *so* incredibly thankful for. After going through a full personal and medical history, talking through my current physical situation/symptoms and where my emotions, feelings and thoughts were at, she discussed treatment options.

She gave me the courtesy of allowing me to be involved in the treatment choice, given that I am a pharmacist. However, because I was so unwell and cognitively I was unable to make any choices or decisions, I completely trusted her and her judgement. Though not first-line therapy, she had prescribed Valdoxan to help induce my sleep and since I had not slept in *weeks,* I thought this was a good option. She also had samples in her practice which meant that I didn't have to take my baby to another place whilst feeling so anxious and inept! So I chose that and hoped for the best.

I remember leaving the appointment, putting Ari in the capsule and then just crying in my car with my whole heart and soul. I fully surrendered to whoever or whatever it was that could help me, to bring me back to myself.

I cried out of exhaustion.

I cried out of fear.

I cried out of frustration.

Yet, I cried out for hope. Hope that this would be the magical fix that I needed so that I could re-enter into my light.

I felt like I had held on for so long and had hit rock bottom, that I needed to get better. I had to for my beautiful boy. No ifs. No buts.

The medications I knew from my pharmacist background can take approximately 1 to 3 weeks to see an improvement, whilst the full effect to be seen can take up to 6 to 8 weeks. I knew I had to be patient. Luckily upon starting, they did allow me to sleep within the first handful of days, which was AMAZING! I remember feeling more rested, though with a heavy head the next day, however a noticeable and grateful change! There was no change in my mood though.

So we waited.

SYDNEY

Thankfully I saw my specialist weekly so I could give feedback as to what was helping and if any changes were seen. There was no change though. By this time, it was early September and Chandi was going to Sydney for a course. Whilst we thought pre-birth that I would be fine to manage on my own by then, unfortunately this wasn't the case. So I decided to go with him to Sydney and stay with my parents, and use the help there whilst I got better. So off to Sydney I went, after Chandi packed all of my bags and organised everything for me and Ari. I found it very overwhelming and my anxiety was hitting the roof. On the outside though, I would look like a picture of a loving mother holding her baby on the plane. Really, I was dying from darkness and suffocation inside.

When I arrived in Sydney, I felt overwhelmed with the love, care and attention that my family gave to me. It had been a few weeks since their return, so it was so nourishing to be near all of my loved ones. I ended up staying there for 6 weeks with Chandi flying back and forth throughout.

Thankfully whilst in Sydney, my Dad was able to get me in to see my Aunty who is a doctor. When we met with her, I spoke about my loop, my inability to make decisions, my feelings, my anxiety and kept asking her if I would get better. Her kindness, calmness yet strength and poise, gave me a stability and confidence to trust in her and to fully surrender into her path and course of treatment, and to just let go.

She prescribed Lexapro, which was first-line therapy at the time, as well as the pill to regulate my hormones after I asked if it may help in returning my hormones back to normal, as I was taking Yasmin previously. She assured me that I would get better. 100 percent better. I was able to stop my Valdoxan, which I was on for just over a month to five weeks by that stage, and begin Lexapro without any washout period. She was an absolute Earth angel who was there for me and supported me when I felt so helpless, misunderstood and so miserably unhappy.

We had my prescription filled and I took the medications immediately. The next morning, I felt really nauseous and quite dizzy. I remember my sister being so excited that I was having a reaction as it meant that it was working. By this point I was hopeful, but I had been so disappointed up until this point, that I didn't know what to believe or expect. I had hope but was not holding onto an idealistic outcome and just went with the flow. I went to sleep as my 'new normal'; not happy, not present, just low, sombre and disconnected self.

RECOVERY

The next morning, 48-hours after taking my new medication when I was in week-11 post-birth, I was woken up by Ari cooing and gurgling in the cot. Normally I would put the covers over my head and cringe with the sound, wishing that it wasn't a new day, or that I could just disappear from this reality. The pit in my stomach as I realised that this was yet another day of the same darkness and despair, normally sent me into a spiral.

Yet, this morning as soon as I heard this gurgling noise from Ari, my eyes opened wide, my head felt clear and I cried in utter joy! I remember saying to Chandi, 'Oh my God, that's *our* baby!'. I knew instantly that the big, dark, heavy body bag that I was wearing had been unzipped and I jumped out of bed and ran to grab Ari!

I cuddled him, held him and felt him on my skin and soul almost for the first time with *absolute* love, connection and so much joy and appreciation!

I just cried and cried and cried! Beautifully warm and heartfelt tears, as I held this gorgeous being that had patiently waited for this moment week after week.

My head felt clear, my mind was pristine, my heart was filled with *so much* emotion and joy that I could literally scream and burst at the seams! I could *feel* emotion again and the clarity was palpably contrasting to what I had endured for those 11 weeks, day in and day out. The way light looked and felt was different. The way I saw life out of my eyes was different. It felt bright. Luminous. Precious. Brighter than anything I had ever seen before.

From that moment at week 11, I considered myself to be fully healed. I was present. I felt whole. I felt complete and so *utterly* in love with my baby that I did not let him go.

My smile returned.

My conversation returned.

My anxiety lifted and disappeared.

My fog was gone.

My eyes had my soul return back into them...and I had returned back into my light.

It was such a stark contrast that it almost had to be seen to be believed. Yet, here I was standing in my real self. It seems almost impossible that a chemical reaction can cause such a *profound* effect on a person. Turn their thought processes inside out and upside down. Turn relationships and connections on their head. From being a bright and bubbly person filled with political correctness and politeness, to be filled with so many crazy thoughts that were articulated to whoever was listening. Yet, with the receptors activated just as I finished my fourth trimester to the week; I had returned back home. The hormonal and biochemical cascade that wreaked havoc in my thoughts, feelings, emotions and life had recalibrated and reached an equilibrium or sparked back, to allow me to think and feel as me. Namita.

The rest of my journey of early motherhood with baby Ari was magical and just as I had imagined it to be, if not *better*. I felt a soul connection to him and I felt so connected to *all* of life. I loved every moment with him. He was so much fun and so fat and cute as I had hoped from my babies! I felt like we had experienced such profound darkness and despair, that through contrast I could *only* savour all the moments of perfection and absolutely devour them all as being sacred and perfect.

All of the sleepless nights, mess, chaos and noise were all there as all parenthood involves, but it was welcomed with gratitude and an awareness, that it is what it is. There was a knowing that with mental health restored there was nothing that was too big or challenging. I welcomed the crying and emotion that came with it, because I knew what feeling no emotion felt like. I welcomed being able to fall asleep and wake when Ari woke, but be able to go straight back to sleep as soon as my head hit the pillow, because I know what no sleep felt like. I welcomed the cuddles because the arms of a baby wrapped around your neck is *the* most magical experience ever, and felt even sweeter upon rising.

I lived with brutal honesty and authenticity about my days and I did not have to pretend they were rainbows and butterflies if they weren't. Yet, on the most part my heart was full and my life felt so amazingly sacred. I was and knew I was completely blessed, because I could have lost all of this had I not stepped into my recovery. I would never have been able to feel that abounding and all transcending love and magic. I would have missed out on all of these divine moments.

How could I not but live in anything other than gratitude and humility?

HEALTH TIP:

WHAT DO I WISH I KNEW BEFORE I HAD CHILDREN?

+ *That it is messy, chaotic and loud most of the time, but the house becomes a home with all of this*

+ *There is no manual. No one has a copy for your child. Trust your instincts and know that you will always make the right decision with the information that you know at the time*

+ *No one has it all figured out! Parenting changes every day as our children grow and evolve, as do we. Go with the flow of it and learn as you go because the landscape is never 'consistent' or 'predictable'*

+ *Sleep whenever you can and never feel guilty about resting your body, mind and soul. These beings can suck the life out of you, so rest when you feel the need to!*

+ *That I would learn a love that I had never known before. I would know what it feels like to have my heart outside of my body and when they run, laugh, smile and joke it would make my heart grow even bigger than I even thought was physically possible*

+ *That we will worry no matter how old they are and will always want the best for them*

+ *That I would need to make space and time for what I enjoy as nothing is ever a 'perfect time' when children are around. We cannot wait until they move out to re-start what we love doing, so do it now, whenever and however you can fit it into your day*

+ *Everything I thought was 'big' or 'important' before children actually is all 'small stuff'. Don't sweat the small stuff and just devour every moment with these gorgeous beings that one day will grow up and no longer need you as much as they do now. You are their whole world and it feels more amazing than anything else on Earth*

31

CHAPTER 2

BABY KAIYAAN

Motherhood with Ari continued to be a magical experience and I loved the amazing time that we had together. We would go to swimming class, music class, Gymbaroo and so many trips to the beach and parks. He was a huge ball of energy and I found myself completely immersed in giving him the very best of me and all of the experiences in life that I could.

When he was 18 months old, we moved from Cairns to Perth for our businesses and it was another exciting chapter in our lives. We met some beautiful friends and had a taste of a bigger city life and all of the range of experiences that we could do together there as a family.

As he grew older and older, I shuddered any time anyone asked when we were having our second baby because for a long time, Ari was going to be an only child. I would blame his intensity and that he was a high energy baby for not being in a hurry. Whilst true, and he still is my wild Ari who tests my patience and boundaries, yet the truth was that I was traumatised and so unbelievably scared that it would happen again. Chandi was ready to have a second child anytime but I held myself back until deep within my heart, I felt like I could handle it if it did happen again.

I had to do *a lot* of inner work navigating through my experience. Journalling my feelings of guilt, shame, embarrassment of that time and how awful I felt putting Ari, my husband, parents, in-laws, siblings and little Ruphus through such an ordeal. I did some amazing work with a lady called Gemma throughout the five years we ended up staying in Perth, and she helped me make so many profound shifts and leaps in my growth. She has the softest, kind and maternal energy that really helped me along my journey. It took me until Ari was three and a half years old before I felt ready to add to our family.

Through my reflection of my first pregnancy and experience, it made me attribute 'logical reasons' and explanations as to *why* I had developed post-natal depression, especially given that I had no underlying history of any anxiety or depression throughout my life. Perhaps it was my Type A personality, my need for control, my scientific logical or 'masculine' mind, I had put it down to *several* factors. Most or all of which I can unequivocally say are *not* the reasons why I developed post-natal depression; which I discovered from conducting my own experiment from pregnancy one to pregnancy two, to be able to safely come up with these conclusions.

Essentially, I blamed my excessive weight gain during pregnancy (and it was truly excessive...mortified!) as a reason for altering my brain biochemistry, so I vowed that the next pregnancy I would not gain as much weight. I blamed that I did stop actively working full-time by 6 months into my pregnancy and that if I had worked right up until 2 weeks before he arrived, that I would not have been so sedentary and that would not have affected my brain biochemistry nor the optimal foetal positioning of Ari.

I blamed the fact that I had an emergency C-section as being the reason that affected my ability to breast feed successfully, and also the trauma of the birth and birth disappointment was what caused my PND. As a result, I then vowed and was adamant that I wanted to try for a VBAC.

I blamed not being prepared with enough of our family nearby prior to going into labour, so I vowed that we would arrange for our family to come in advance and be ready. I blamed the fact that we lived in a small and dark apartment and that is what contributed to my dark and depressed state. So we bought a big, bright and light filled home in beautiful Applecross in Perth. You name it, I used my logic to place blame and reason for causing the PND.

In hindsight I am grateful that I did change all of the variables from the first pregnancy to the next, because I can stand here confidently and say that having polar opposite factors within two pregnancies caused the exact *same outcome*. Aside from having an epidural in both births, there was nothing else that was replicated, yet exactly on day 5 post-partum I sank into my post-natal depression and exactly at week 11 I regained 'consciousness' again.

Nothing I did had caused it. *Nothing*.

How liberating that felt for me and still is to this day.

I can relinquish any guilt or blame that I had put onto myself and just move forward with freedom, knowing that I *could not* control the outcome, no matter what master orchestrator I thought I was. It is in my DNA, my biochemistry, the blue-print of who I am when I was created.

I digress! When we finally felt ready to embark upon welcoming another beautiful soul into our hearts and home, I was *beyond* blessed to fall pregnant on the first month of trying. I was *so* ecstatic yet shocked as to how quickly it transpired but I knew that this baby didn't want to miss their chance, given how long I waited with hesitation...so got in quick before I changed my mind!

My pregnancy was much harder this time around and I was vomiting ten times a day from 4pm all through the night. I was vomiting so much that I burst blood vessels in my cheeks and had to have a fluid drip a couple of times at the GP. My *amazing* obstetrician gave me Ondansetron which was the strongest medication option, but it still did not stop my vomiting. Thankfully at the 18-week mark it miraculously just stopped; which I was beyond grateful for!

As I promised myself, I was super mindful with my weight gain and was very careful about what I ate. I did my pregnancy yoga class once a week and then would do it at home throughout the rest of the week. I used to still go to the gym a few times a week and walk Ari to school. In the end, I had only gained 13 kilograms which was almost one third of the weight I gained the first time! I was super proud of my efforts and felt empowered knowing that weight gain was no longer a variable in the context of causing my PND, as I had done everything in my power to keep that within reasonable limits.

I was focussed on having a VBAC from the outset, so I enrolled myself in the Hypnobirthing program and listened to the beautiful tracks religiously. I focussed on the beautiful and calm VBAC that I wanted throughout my entire pregnancy. I was mindful of how I sat on my bed, whilst driving and the optimum foetal positioning of the baby. It made the last part of pregnancy very uncomfortable as I sat with my tummy held forward instead of reclined, just so I knew without a shadow of a doubt that I had done everything humanly possible to support a natural delivery this time around. In hindsight I wasted a lot of time and energy focusing incessantly on being in the right position, that I could have just relaxed in my pregnancy and enjoyed my freedom and life before a second baby joined us. Hindsight is wonderful...but does not change a thing!

I joined a local ABA (Australian Breastfeeding Association) group so that I had people I could contact and knew, should I have any trouble breastfeeding this time around. Being prepared and organised allowed me to feel empowered and that I was setting all my ducks in order ready for whatever was thrown at me.

I spoke in depth to my obstetrician (who I absolutely *loved* by the way!) and midwives about my post-natal depression last time. I explained how I normally feel and the contrast with how I felt at the time of my illness, that I would be able to identify if I felt off again. I also felt supported knowing that everyone knew what we were dealing with upfront. I also said that the Lexapro was what worked last time and if I need it again then I have no shame or reservation with going on it as soon as any signs presented this time around. I've got this, I thought.

We also booked tickets for my parents to come at 38-weeks should an elective C-section be booked in for me or if I went into labour early. They would stay for four weeks and then Chandi's parents would fly in as my parents went back. I felt so comfortable knowing that our family would be near us and we were not naïve as to what tremendous support we needed after having a baby. I will be forever grateful as to how much of themselves they all gave to us.

What is interesting upon reflection, is that though I had done a lot of healing work, there was still *so* much control associated with the outcome. I didn't fully surrender or trust in the process and essentially used my body as a laboratory conducting my own experiment with my own hypotheses and theories behind it. *True* surrender would allow the outcome to happen organically irrespective of what I *wanted* it to look like. Yet, at least now there was no room for any 'should have', 'could have' thinking so for that I am grateful for my steadfast focus. A true scientist living my experiment out!

My pregnancy was amazing once the vomiting stopped, and we found out that we were having another little boy, though I was adamant that I was carrying a girl. His energy felt so feminine, soft and gentle which was so different to Ari, which immediately felt very masculine. To be fair, Kaiyaan *is* a very gentle, soft, delicate and sensitive boy, who is the feminine touch that our household needed. He has a very special place in all of our hearts and so my intuition of his femininity was accurate. I also had Reiki with beautiful Gemma once a month throughout my pregnancy, which became a beautiful connective activity that I looked forward to each time.

My obstetrician was not against trying for a VBAC but was more encouraging of an elective caesarean. He did however let me see how I felt as we progressed. I was having weekly acupuncture for my fluid retention as I didn't want to resemble the Elephant Man this pregnancy! By week 36 the acupuncturist started slowly preparing my body for labour with my sole intention of having a VBAC.

I also started induction massage at 37 weeks to slowly encourage my body to prepare for labour, which we ramped up at 38 weeks. I continued with my yoga, Hypnobirthing, exercise and thankfully at 39 weeks, I started to go into labour.

BIRTH

The morning I went into labour I was having cramps from around 7am. I started getting contractions and so Chandi raced home from work and we were in the hospital by 11am. I listened to my Hypnobirthing tracks and my favourite singer Snatam Kaur and I was in my 'zone'. I was 10cm by close to 3pm and Kaiyaan was born at 3.26pm after a beautiful, seamless and magical VBAC.

I felt so much admiration and gratitude for my body. I felt so unbelievably empowered.

I felt *so* much love and emotion.

I immediately felt connected to him and absolutely savoured this divine being. *Every* cell of him.

I was filled with adrenaline and oxytocin. Ari meeting Kaiyaan for the first time was so beautiful and I will remember the emotion I felt forever in that moment. It was *so* divinely special and perfect.

The time in the hospital was amazing. I still did have trouble with latching Kaiyaan but I did not ask every nurse in the entire hospital to watch on this time! He was naturally more calm and serene so I felt better able to try myself and hoped for the best. My supply was low and on the second day a nurse came in with my Motilium (Domperidone), which is a medication to help stimulate the production of milk that I had discussed with my OB, given my horror experience with Ari. It works by blocking dopamine, the neurotransmitter notoriously involved in pleasure, euphoria and motivation, in order to enhance Prolactin which is responsible for milk production, in a very simple breakdown. My gut reaction when she offered it to me was just to wait and see how I went as it was still early on in our breastfeeding journey. Yet, when she was walking out the door for *some* reason I ignored this internal feeling, I stopped her and decided that I would start taking it. I slowly increased my dosage as prescribed as the days progressed, as I desperately wanted to breastfeed my beautiful boy.

I continued having issues with latching so tried multiple techniques to no avail. I will admit that the recovery after a natural delivery was *so* much easier, and moving my body to feed him was much easier and less painful than after having my emergency C-section. I started to pump on the last day to boost my supply and syringe feed him as somehow I was having the same trouble with feeding him as I had with Ari. Thankfully though in the hospital, I was feeling myself and was able to handle this feeding choreography that seemed to be a consistent theme.

Going home on day three was a magical and special experience and one that I will never forget. We were *so* happy, so in love and so proud that I was doing well, especially compared to last time where I was riddled with anxiety on our way home. Our dog Ruphus was so excited to see us and him meeting Kaiyaan was such a beautiful and priceless experience.

I was home. My heart was happy and full and we were in absolute bliss.

Day 4 rolled on in and I woke up and I started to feel the pins and needles on my chest and intrinsically knew that my anxiety was returning. It felt like an uncomfortable stabbing and hot type of pain on my chest. There was no denying that it felt exactly how it started last time and literally it had come on overnight.

I brought my Dad and Chandi into our room and I sat them down explaining that I was feeling the anxiety slowly creeping in again. I wanted to share how I was feeling with them as part of being open and honest from the outset. They were extremely supportive and so proud that I spoke up immediately, and they were on standby should anything escalate now that we were all on guard.

That first day I was still able to function well and kept busy with the boys. I played with Ari and Kaiyaan and was able to push through it hoping that it would pass. I still felt like myself for the most part. Breastfeeding was still not working for me and I continued to express after trying to latch him on, but felt like we were not able to choreograph our dance very well together, but continued taking Motilium to boost my supply.

I was unable to sleep again at all that night as I was riddled with my anxiety. Pins and needles became hotter and sharper and my mind raced around incessantly. Kaiyaan would wake every two to three hours, but I was wired and up ready for him dreading the next feed and feeling like my spiral was gaining momentum.

I rose out of bed that next day and the dreaded day 5 had arrived. Like a flick of a switch overnight, I had re-entered my heavy black suit with a huge dark cloud over my head. My smile had gone, my mood was dark and sombre and I had gone from a happy, vibrant, vivacious and joyous being into a sad, dark, almost soulless person who had lost any sense of emotion or connection.

I had gone from 100 to 0 in 24 hours flat. Nothing had changed except the course of time and I was no longer there.

The essence of me; my joy, emotion and heart had disappeared into the ether.

I didn't have to articulate with anybody as to what had changed overnight. Suffice to say when Chandi and my parents looked at me, they knew they were looking at a blank canvas. My eyes were empty and my soul had vanished.

They knew undeniably that I had left the building.

My ability to do my normal activities and functions with confidence, strength and power were *immediately* replaced with doubt, inability to make a decision, to take action or know what to do. Simple and basic tasks like selecting an outfit to wear was impossible. The process of expressing milk had *instantly* become too difficult and seemingly a mammoth task, though I was completely fine with the whole process the night before. I was unable to give direction to my Mum of what to make Ari for lunch, or be able to take charge as I normally do.

I went from the leader of the home into a vacant guest. Overnight.

I don't think any of us realised the severity of the state that I had entered into because it happened so rapidly and so profoundly. It had come with full force this time around. From the very outset I had fallen into having strong ideations right away and thought of all the ways in which I could leave this all behind. Logic cannot understand how this can happen so abruptly yet, it truly did. Only time had ticked on by and tipped me on the edge.

I saw no hope.

I saw no way out.

I felt like I was in a different world. Instantly.

The darkness and horrible thoughts I was thinking and feeling were so unlike me and in stark contrast to the euphoric state I felt just 48 hours earlier. I am still to this day shocked as to what a huge impact that the biochemical cascade of neurotransmitters and hormones in my system had set off, simply from giving birth. The hormonal shift caused an eruption of a truly deep, dark depression and was the cause of all my warped and intrusive thoughts.

That day my parents and Chandi discussed about the best course of action as there was no avoiding the profound change in my biochemistry overnight. We called my Aunty who had helped me last time and explained what I was feeling and what was happening and she liaised with my GP to begin a course of Lexapro straight away, as that was what had given beautiful results last time. Then we waited.

I had started medication on day 6 in the hope of beginning straight away, so that I would return to healthy functioning much sooner. Each moment I could see the anticipation of everyone waiting to see this miraculous recovery that I had made within 48 hours of starting it last time; though it was 10 weeks later and after I had already tried another agent.

Our intentions were pure, directed and one of taking action which we *all* should be proud of.

Unfortunately, day after day passed and there was no improvement. I could not sleep at all. Not a wink. Not even for a second. My brain was hard wired on full anxiety mode, major pins and needles on my chest to the point of it feeling like the heaviest, hottest weight on me. My head was racing and I could not talk about anything else except my repetitive loop. I kept saying 'What have we done? Why did we think it would be different? It was better before. What were we thinking? Everything was easy before, why have we made our lives so complicated?'.

That was all I could think. All I could talk about.

It presented in the *exact* same way as last time, except it was further and deeper.

The anxiety was actually physically painful and I would dread night-time the most. I had no distractions so the stabbing feeling felt so much more acute. My mouth was so dry and my appetite had jumped out the window as I would imagine myself doing time and time again. Repetitively.

My parents and Chandi listened with patience and compassion to my fixation on my loop to start with, despite what I was saying being *so* painful and hurtful to listen to, with this most perfect, healthy and amazing baby in our home. Our dream baby.

They offered kindness and support without judgement. They listened. They were there. Every single moment.

I am *so* grateful for my parents, Chandi and his parents once they did arrive, that between them they did all of the cooking, looked after the laundry, all of Ari's meals, taking him to school, playing with him, looking after Kaiyaan whilst I tried to get some sleep or rest. They did *everything*.

Everyone's focus like last time was to allow me to get some sleep and perhaps the medication could work better and my recovery would be possible. I was in our room with Kaiyaan but Chandi would wake up with him all through the night in the hope that I would rest and not have that pressure to look after him. In the morning when Ari would run into our room at 5.30/6am, Chandi, after not sleeping at all with Kaiyaan, would go and play with Ari. I would just stay in bed in a foetal position, find someone to listen to my loop or just sit there silent with no ability to have a conversation about anything else.

Every day I sat blankly looking into space ruminating through all of my dysfunctional thoughts. Hours would go by without me even realising it or I would find someone to latch my claws into to listen to my loop. I was like a broken record and could say the same thing hundreds of times within the hour and articulated every single thought I had in my incessantly racing mind.

I would message my sister one message after the next, after the next, after the next and pour (or rather dump) all of my feelings onto her. I would then do the same with my brother, then Chandi and then my parents. As soon as I made eye contact, out of my mouth would flow the verbal diarrhoea. One to the other. To the next.

I am so grateful for all my family support staying with us at home (my parents first then my in-laws once my parents went back), having Chandi at home, in Sydney with my sister and brother, as there is *no* way that this boat would not have sunk if we did not have the life support and raft of our family at that time. *Not* a chance in the world.

This is the absolute truth of the situation I was in.

My admiration for you ladies who are single, or do not have support, is *endless*. I can only imagine the reality of the pressures that are on your shoulders, so I *implore* you to reach out for any support from friends, family or to start the conversation with your GP to arrange access to support services in order to assist you. There is no need to suffer through this alone. This could be a matter of life and death, and is so unbelievably essential.

We had child health nurses visit and lactation consultants from the hospital came to visit us at home. I was continuing expressing whilst trying to feed him and despite all of the help, it just was not working at all. I even went to a local pharmacy that had a lactation consultant but I felt like I was having a panic attack in the room. It was in a small enclosed space with the door shut and I felt like the room was closing in on me. I felt like I couldn't breathe. I felt like I was suffocating, Kaiyaan was screaming his lungs out and I felt like just running out of there. It was a horrible feeling that I still can remember so clearly even to this day.

I kept taking the Motilium until day 10 when I thought again, after chatting with the child health nurse, that the breastfeeding hormones *could* be what was making me feel that way, so stopped taking the medication and stopped expressing and changed over to formula.

I had made more peace with it this time rather than hammering myself with guilt. My thoughts and fog were so much deeper this time, that it didn't allow room to bring in extra elements of emotion. I couldn't physically keep up with the expressing and I dreaded doing it all every 2 hours, and the disconnection and resentment grew and grew as the days went on. Switching to formula was the right decision for me at that stage.

We continued like this for a few weeks with no signs of improvement, anxiety ravaging my body and not eating or sleeping *at all*. I had someone near me at all times. Everyone knew how delicate this situation was and what a strong hold this post-natal depression had on me this time around. On consultation with my GP and Aunty, we ended up doubling my dose of Lexapro and hoped again that this shift would be enough to make a change in how I was feeling. My Aunty was available for me whenever I needed her and her love, support and encouragement to keep on going allowed me the courage to keep fighting another day. I am proud that we made additions to my medication management based on seeing no change. We also had added Endep (Amitriptyline) at around this point to help with my sleep and mood; with the only noticeable change being that it caused an even drier mouth than I already had, with no profound improvement.

At least we all knew this time *what* was causing my dysfunctional thoughts and behaviour, whereas last time it was *all* brand new and we had no idea what was happening. There was an element of disappointment that it happened again and a sense of fatigue. Almost like a Covid fatigue; where again we didn't know the exact end-point and the pressure to keep fronting up day after day with no change was *exhausting*; both physically and emotionally.

However, they all held and carried me throughout this entire journey. Whether it was Chandi and my parents or in-laws helping me at home (all flying to be with us from Sydney), reassuring me that I would get through this and allowing me the time and space to heal, without them putting any pressure on me personally. Or whether it was my sister and brother in Sydney who listened to me non-stop, replied to my endless and incessant messages, who took time away from their children and work to be available for me 24/7. Though I didn't realise it at the time, my sister had to pull herself away from her business just so that she could be available for me whenever

I needed her, which was all the time, as the strain on her body to do both was physically impossible. My brother would give me kind advice and support and would check in on how we were *all* doing day after day with so much love and compassion. They *all* breathed life into me and kept me holding on.

Just like last time, I had clutched my claws into each and every one of them and it would have been all-consuming for them with fear and worry about my wellbeing and possible future, as well as engulfing all of *them* even though they were not the ones who physically had the baby. Though everyone helped in different ways, the enormous strain that I placed on all of my family during this time I am *so* mindfully aware of, and my heart fills with sadness and guilt that I caused all of this. Though I am so unbelievably grateful. I will forever feel indebted for the profound effect that it had on their time, life and health. All of them.

My primal knowledge kept me holding on for my children. I had this inner awareness that I could not leave them behind without their mother and it was *this* knowing that kept me holding on each hour, even though it felt *impossible*. Yet, despite this innate knowing, my connection with Ari had disappeared too as I genuinely didn't know how I interacted with him before. I hardly spoke to him except for very robotic disconnected type questions after school but he knew the essence of me was missing and was getting *so* frustrated with me. He was reacting with anger and he couldn't even look at me without anger or disappointment; and I do not blame him at all.

This poor innocent four year old was dealing with concepts so *far* out of his understanding.

That disconnection was with Ruphus our dog too. He would not come anywhere near me and I wouldn't know how to interact with him. This is the only way I can describe how it felt, which sounds so ludicrous as to how one loses their connection instantly? I truly felt like my soul and heart had left my body and I had no ability to connect with anyone.

After some time of not being able to fall asleep in our room, we thought I may have uninterrupted sleep in Ari's room and since Kaiyaan was on formula now, Chandi completely took over the nights so that I could hopefully sleep. I would lie on an air mattress in Ari's room tossing and turning and not sleeping a wink. I would be festering through my incessant thoughts of regret, my ruminating thoughts that continued to become darker and saw no hope or way out of it night after night. The physical anxiety was uncomfortable and I *dreaded* nights so unbelievably much.

Ari would wake up in the morning, take one look at me on the floor and run out of the door not saying a word, even if our eyes connected. I would lie in bed unable to move or get up. I felt so bogged down in my depression like I was buried in sand or suffocating in a zipped bag with no air coming in, so I would cover my body with the blanket hoping to make this all disappear.

Motivation zero. Connection to life double zero.

My beautiful Kaiyaan. My heart rips with sadness that I could leave this beautiful divine baby in the hands of others when all he would have craved and wanted was to be held by his mother in her warm loving embrace. I did hold him and care for him of course, but my heart was not switched on. I would change his nappy and feed him but I would just be going through the motions and not truly connecting to any of it at all.

How could I treat this beautiful boy, my soul baby like this? Even as I write this, my heart aches and cries that my beautiful boy who makes my blood jump for joy now, had to suffer like this alone; and I was the mother who needed to give him the love and connection he needed in this big, wide world.

Those weeks of feeling *so* disconnected to my children is the most heart-breaking part of PND. It is the most horrendous reality of post-natal depression, that has such a *huge* impact on these innocent children who crave love and connection from their mother more than anything else. This illness took that away from me and stripped me of enjoying and connecting with my most amazing boys for *all* those weeks. It is time and moments that I can *never ever* get back.

It is the cruelest illness to cause such feelings between a mother and her children. The cruelest.

They didn't deserve that. I didn't deserve that.

You do not deserve that.

Yet, the knowledge that <u>this is</u> the illness speaking and acting out, and by sharing with you that I sought treatment, it may help you to come out of this sense of disconnection. My hope is that you too can enter into that connection and love with your children after reading about my experiences.

The love and connection *will* come back. I absolutely promise you and it *feels* AMAZING.

Every breath I take has my children etched within it now. It is actually as the cliché says of watching your heart beating on the outside when you look at them. The sooner you take that step forward, the sooner you will feel your heart centre again and step into *your* joy with *your* children.

A few weeks of this waiting and holding on had passed, and with weeks of sleepless nights, there was no doubt that Chandi's patience was waning and he was getting frustrated by the whole situation. My Aunty had told him that it was vital that everyone stopped listening to my loop because by talking about it, it consolidated the loop and would strengthen its place in my thought process and belief system, making it harder for me to heal and recover.

I, at the time did not know this, so felt like Chandi had shut down completely and I felt like he didn't understand what I was saying or how I was feeling. Especially since he had gone from listening to me 24/7 with so much empathy and kindness and then suddenly not listening to it at all, it felt very isolating and I felt very much alone and confused when that happened. There were a few communication breakdowns about this handling of my speaking about the loop and whilst everyone wanted me to get better, this underlying tension and strain did weigh on my shoulders and was a heavy feeling in my heart, or whatever was left of it during that time.

All around it *is* a hard situation and a *very* stressful time. It was palpable. The reality is, a time like this becomes like a pressure cooker for everyone involved. Add in emotions, sleep deprivation and seeing life through different filters; it is no wonder that there can be a huge strain on all relationships through a crisis like this; and it is truly a crisis.

It actually is a situation where everyone feels worried, helpless and out of control, as no one can predict or know the exact way out and *does* test the patience of everyone closest to you. I am not writing this to add any further guilt or pressure onto you. Not at all. Rather, by being honest and raw about the reality of the tension and strain that *can* arise through differing opinions and perspectives of those closest to you; as to how they feel it should be handled; what could be done better; who can do more, or who should do less...is to hopefully help you see that it *is* a natural repercussion, it can happen and *if* it is happening with you and your family, then please do not feel alone. You are *not* alone and you will get through this time.

It is important to share though, that the pressure and undue stress that this type of contention can bring to an already delicate situation, is added darkness for the mother. Whilst I was not cognisant, nor connected to my heart-centre to feel emotion, I still was able to recognise that any of this extra heaviness did not serve me and my recovery *at all*. Time is the greatest healer, and I can only stand in my power of recognising how this illness debilitated *me* and *my connection* with myself and my boys. I could have left this all behind twice and I denied my beautiful boys the connection to their mother during that time, which they didn't deserve...and *this* is the *true essence* of this illness and everything additional is noise.

My hope for all of you women, is that everyone sees the mother as the patient that requires synergistic working together to lead you towards healing. Everyone holding hands. Everyone holding your hand. My hope is that everyone could see life through one common filter. Through the same lens. My hope is that there are no extra layers of emotion and heaviness for you to sift through. Not there at all. Not hanging as extra weight on your shoulders and weighing heavily on your heart. This is possibly idealism at its finest but if possible to achieve, this would be the best possible scenario in a crisis like this.

I know in my heart of hearts that life is what it is and I have made peace with all aspects of this in my life and my healing. To step forward into my learnings from it, and that is the space where my power lies. I am eternally grateful with *every cell* in my being that I had strong, amazing, heart-centred husband and family members giving me *all* of themselves in my recovery, and I will always remember the time, effort and life they missed out on just to help me in my darkest hour and in every minute of each hour. Always. If you have this available too, then how blessed we are indeed.

We were in contact with my obstetrician also quite frequently who was *so* incredibly supportive when I explained what was happening and he would call me daily to check in on how I was feeling and to make sure that I was OK. It was like speaking to a friend, I felt that much empathy from him. He brought forward my 6-week appointment and looked after me so delicately and well. I am so eternally grateful for him and the way he went above and beyond, during the darkest period of my life and I will be *forever* grateful.

He organised for me to visit a psychologist in the same private hospital and I was able to get into her within a few days of speaking to him. Ironically she lived a few houses down from us in Perth and I saw her around school, but never knew who she was until I needed her but would see her all the time after that...synchronicity!

When I saw her I was an absolute mess. Crying, going over my repetitive loop, discussing the stress of the situation and she listened without judgement and an open ear and heart. She said that we needed to get the brain chemistry right and until we found the right solution and combination then we wouldn't be able to make breakthroughs with other things. She was definitely another one of my Earth angels and I hold her in such a high regard in my heart and soul for the compassion, kindness, strength and care that she demonstrated to me and my family, at a time when I had given up *all* hope. I leant on her with all of my heart and she really did help lighten my load and the hope she filled me with, carried me forward one day at a time.

It was now late October and I had a referral to a local psychiatrist to help, as it was becoming evident that all of my medication was not working despite being on it for at least 7 weeks. However, the doctor was fully booked until December. Chandi and I both separately had called so many specialists from a Google search and everyone was either not taking new patients or were fully booked until the new year. I felt so helpless and exhausted both mentally and physically. I felt like this was all so futile and that I would be stuck feeling like this forever and saw no light at the end of the tunnel.

So I went back to my GP for a referral to someone else and she sent through a referral to The Elizabeth Clinic which specialises in antenatal and post-natal care for both mothers and their children. She said they were usually very busy but I *pleaded* with her that it was urgent and if she could do her best for someone to see me. Thankfully seeing the dire position that I was in, they called me and I managed to get an appointment within a few weeks for which I was *so* utterly thankful and relieved.

I remember feeling so nervous and anxious about seeing this specialist but I also had hit rock bottom and felt so *utterly exhausted* from this whole situation that I desperately needed to get better. Deep within my soul, I knew that I could not go on for a moment longer feeling this way.

No sleep. Not even for a minute.

No food. Maybe a mouthful or two per day at most.

Constant anxiety that physically *hurt*. Intensely. Like knives cutting into the depths of my soul. Making it feel like I could not breathe.

Thick, dark and heavy fog that suffocated my brain; unable to function in the most basic tasks.

Staring blankly into the abyss of space for hours on end...looking as lost and vacant as I felt.

Empty eyes. Empty heart. Empty soul. No smile. Nothing to say except for my loop.

Tensions raw and palpable...Wanting to disappear and end all of this torture and hell right here on planet Earth.

I saw no point, and that everyone's lives would be easier without my mess and the heaviness that I was causing.

When I met with her, I was a babbling mess and told her everything I was thinking and feeling and she listened. Without judgement. With patience. She was a lot more 'alpha' in nature than anyone else thus far, and she told me exactly her analysis of my situation; which was that my 'thoughts were extremely sticky and muddy'. Yet, she took control of the situation and created a very specific and concrete plan to move forward.

I needed that.

I loved that.

I felt a confidence in her strength, her experience, her ability to understand what I was saying. She was the one who gave me the best explanation of what I was experiencing. Up until that time I had no idea what on earth was wrong with me!

She explained that from pregnancy to breastfeeding our hormones within our bodies drop suddenly by 100 times in level. This profound change sets off a switch in the brain that can pull mothers off the tracks like a train and we are just running off the tracks with our thoughts. We need to turn that switch back the other way so that the train can return back to its path. She said that this level affects around 1 percent of the population, but she assured me that I *would* get better.

She gave me a solid plan of how to wean off my current medications and how to slowly start my new course of medication, which was Pristiq. She did prescribe some anti-anxiety medication should I need it when I was doing the weaning and starting the process, which I did not use but mentally I felt armed if it was required. I left feeling optimistic in her taking the reins and steered me in a direction where I didn't have to make any decisions but just do as I was told. I was hopeful and so utterly relieved for getting an appointment with her especially since everywhere else had such long waiting times! I felt like I could almost breathe again, as if this was the right puzzle piece that I was needing.

During week 10 post-birth, I started the weaning process immediately and to be honest I didn't have any side effects at all. I still wasn't sleeping but that wasn't new. I did it over a course of a week and then gradually started my new medication. I felt a bit dizzy with the Pristiq but nothing too profound.

Like any other night, I went to sleep in Ari's room except this time I did *actually* sleep. I dreamt of my Grandmother, who was very ill with cancer in the UK where my parents wanted to go to visit her, but were too worried about me to leave the country. I dreamt that she was tailgating me in Perth and speeding behind me and I remember thinking, what is she doing in Perth? I remember waking up from this dream just as the sun was rising and I opened my eyes and felt a clarity, a clearness and as though the heavy fog had completely lifted off my head and my entire body. It was like someone overnight had unzipped this black suffocating and heavy body suit and allowed me to walk into my true self again.

I lay there for a few moments knowing and feeling within my being that I had returned and that I felt like me again.

It was then that Ari, who had not uttered a word to me or looked at me for the previous ten weeks, crawled into my air mattress on the floor with me. He held me and started singing this Noongar song, an Indigenous song, that I had heard him perform at school for Mother's Day whilst I was pregnant. It went *'Baby you are my heart, baby you are my heart, baby you are my heart, my star, my love, my life'*...and I cried warm, beautiful, joyful tears as I held him.

I *felt* the love. My heart could *feel* again and the darkness had been lifted. The emotions I could actually *feel* again and whilst I didn't even have to articulate anything, Ari intrinsically knew that I was different that morning and came and held me. I felt something so divine and magical in that moment and I also felt completely like myself, and I was so intensely relieved!

I believe my Grandmother came to me as she knew what I was going through and came to check in whilst she was transitioning. I felt her support and her watching over me in that moment.

I ran with Ari into our bedroom where Chandi and Kaiyaan were still asleep but I knew that Chandi would be so relieved and happy to hear that I had miraculously returned back into my body! I jumped into the bed and said that I felt like me again and I saw him smile and he gave me the biggest hug. All three of us lay in the bed holding each other and Kaiyaan was still sleeping in his bassinet.

It was pure perfection and there was *so* much beauty and joy in that moment that I never wanted it to end.

I held them feeling them closely as if I had never held them before, and my heart felt like it could burst at the seams with how grateful and happy I felt.

I had returned home, back to my light. I was back to being connected with my heart-centre which had been completely disconnected. It felt like the air looked, felt and smelt differently and my home shone as if this cloud had gone and the glasses I was looking out of were completely clear and free from debris.

I felt *so* much relief, so much lightness and joy in that moment and when Kaiyaan woke up, I held him and smelt him and devoured every morsel of skin on him and just cried with *so* many emotions.

Gratitude. Happiness. Joy.

Guilt.

Feelings of lost time with my baby boy that I could never ever get back. Eleven arduous and painful weeks where we all suffered and most importantly, my sweet little innocent boy who would have craved beyond anything in the world to have *his mummy* hold him and tell him how much she loved him.

I felt a sadness for the pain that I had caused and yet, pure presence and a heart connection with him and a vow to give my boys the very best of myself from *this* moment on. To cherish this journey of motherhood and to be there in all the ways I could, to give them the best life possible. That moment was like giving birth all over again and yet, *so* much sweeter, because I wouldn't have to endure that pain again as I knew that I had returned.

It was a hugely distinct and obvious return back to myself when the switch clearly came back on. The switch had a definite and obvious switch off and the switch back on was so obvious too.

Once that biochemistry had buzzed me back into life, I felt like my equilibrium was restored and I felt like me again. All of me. The best of me.

I was so grateful for the medication that restored my biochemistry, as otherwise who knows what the alternative could have been. My children may not have a mother. My husband may be a widow, my parents without their youngest child and my siblings without their youngest sister. I may not have been here to recount my tale and to help others recognise their pain and to move towards their recovery.

However, with the strain that ensued from my illness, whilst I was joyous and everyone was too; there was an element of PTSD for the others involved because miraculously I had returned overnight yet, their trauma was raw. I understand that completely and I acknowledge all of what that may look and feel like. The PTSD is real and can recur or pop up when one least expects it. It is no doubt *all* part of the process and I acknowledge it with compassion and appreciate that *time* is the greatest healer of all things. One cannot enter the depths of the trenches in a war, drag everyone into it and not expect a recovery period to be necessary and I humbly acknowledge and allow space and time for that...for all of it x

The rest of my motherhood journey with Kaiyaan, like with Ari, was *pure* joy and happiness. The days were filled with an abundance of love and joy. Riddled with mess, sleepless nights, chaos that all parenthood involves. Yet, with my mental health returned, I could handle anything and do everything. I said *yes* to life; *all* of life. Every moment with my boys felt *so sacred* and I devoured it and still do to this day, savour every embrace, every smile and *every* moment of unconditional love that occurs.

It is through the contrast of how dark, desolate and alone I felt during that time that I am able to appreciate just how amazing I feel with my mental health restored to all of its glory. The contrast is undeniable and I can feel just how polar opposite each state of being felt.

I am filled with gratitude that my heart can feel every ounce of feeling, whatever it may be; happy, sad, frustrated, hurt, joy and everything in between.

I am so grateful to my boys for their patience and unconditional love. They waited for me to return back to my true self and the resilience they demonstrated humbles me every day. The way they forgave me instantly and were genuinely just *so* happy that I had returned, have been my biggest teachers for how pure *unconditional* love is. The unconditional love between mother and child is there always, and whilst I denied them that emotion in those early 11 weeks, they showed me how possible it is to have access to it at *any point* upon our healing. It is *never ever* too late.

They are truly my *greatest teachers*.

Upon healing, I wanted to live life as fully as I could with the knowledge and awareness that tomorrow is not promised to any of us. I began removing my mask and being truly authentic with all of my relationships and being so raw and honest with all of my experiences, so much more than recovering after Ari. I no longer felt the need to hide the essence of me when it had been taken away from me overnight. I will never take for granted my ability to use my voice now that I have it restored. To stand into my power and to live *my* life with unbridled enthusiasm.

I love connecting with all people that I meet and love being open with my experience in the hope of inspiring others to remove their mask, and feel the ability to be comfortable in sharing whatever it is that they need to.

I am proud of the strength within me that held on, spoke up and still held on despite nothing being a 'quick' fix.

I am proud that I no longer feel the weight of anyone's judgement or perception of me or my experience.

I am proud that I am using this knock down as an anchor to help other women to show them that returning to their light and health *is* possible and to scream it from the rooftops that recovery IS available to you. I want to support you throughout your journey of healing.

I am proud that I am not allowing my war-wound to weigh me down but to heal the wounds of others.

I am proud that I am here and can help shine the light on a condition that is filled with so much darkness.

When Kaiyaan was 4 months old, almost immediately after I had recovered, I started studying Homeopathy online. It didn't resonate with my soul as to truly connecting with the modality, yet it was a stepping stone in allowing me to then to begin my journey in studying Ayurveda.

Upon my first few course sessions, Ayurveda gave me so many levels of understanding of our body, mind and spirit connection and truly explained my post-natal depression in another way that I had not seen before. It allowed me to understand an ancient practice that could explain and appreciate the huge fall into my illness during this '4th trimester'; and it truly was the exact amount of time for me. I devoured the content and loved every second with my beautiful teacher, Neerja from Ayurveda Awareness, who I felt so incredibly nurtured by.

It allowed me to look at life with new eyes, yet again, and what I saw was a connection to all of life. I apply the principles in all that I do. What I take in through my senses, my lifestyle, my nutrition and cooking, the way I tailor meals, sounds and activities to best support the different souls living at home. It has been truly revolutionary for me and I genuinely feel like I have a far greater mindfulness and awareness into how I live my life and am aware of the 'cause and effect' relationship so much more.

I went on to learn more tools to help support women with post-natal depression in studying through the Infant Massage Information Service (IMIS) in Sydney to become a PMC (Paediatric Massage Consultant) and CIMI (Certified Infant Massage Instructor). These learnings have been pivotal in offering tools to help mothers in their journey of healing and I wished that I had this knowledge prior to having my own children, as perhaps it would have lessened my symptoms or allowed for a speedier recovery. I feel like this knowledge into infant massage and the plethora of benefits that it provides, to both the mother and baby has deepened my awareness into *how many* tools we do have available to us, in order to help us through our healing journey of PND. I am so grateful to Heidi McLoughlin for her beautiful training and knowledge that she gave to me so that I can help spread the use of this modality far and wide.

I am continuing my education in Ayurvedic Yoga teaching and to become an Ayurveda Lifestyle Consultant through an Ayurvedic centre, Aligning Health Retreat in Bendigo, Victoria with an amazing teaching team that I am thoroughly enjoying. My hope is that I can bring as many tools to help navigate women through their journeys as possible. This is now my life's journey and purpose.

As a result of my experiences, I strive to live my truth for my boys and they drive me to always become better, to heal my inner wounds, my layers that no longer serve me and mindsets that are outdated, limiting and restrictive so that I continue to be the best version of myself for them.

It was through the introduction by my sister to the 'portal of pain' theory by Dr Shefali that explained and made me understand that by hitting *absolute* rock bottom; it was this in and of itself that allowed for my cracks to widen and to connect to the true inner being that was there my entire life. Arriving to the trenches of darkness, not due to anything within my control, has only allowed me to devour and savour every part of life upon rising and to heal all aspects of myself that needed a warm, *nourishing* embrace.

Perhaps this shaking up of my absolute core, has allowed for the deepest healing and awakening that could never have been possible without my boys' presence and guiding light.

I remember having drinks with a lady and openly sharing my journey with her, which was the first time I had shared it with *anyone* except for my family and very close friends. Unfortunately, she shuddered and said that was the thing she was most scared of with more babies and that was it. Silence.

I felt like I had shared my most sacred and deep secret, which was actually very raw at that moment still. Her reaction was not one of openness or holding space for me to be vulnerable. However, my hope is that we *can* create the space for you to share in a way that is *only* received with support and understanding and in a way that you feel *truly* honoured and respected. No longer do I want people to think that PND is a sign of weakness and simply that as mothers we are not coping. Not coping is a *side effect* or symptom of the biochemical imbalance, that does not discriminate.

I want to be clear that this is *real*. It takes people's lives. It causes suffering beyond anything I can *truly* articulate well enough. It affects generations within the one family and the support needs to be given _right now_. Women are the divine gatekeepers into the world, our creators and our nurturers. If I think of what this world would have been like without my Kaiyaan in it, if I had been too traumatised after Ari to have a second child; I know that the world would not have this most beautiful boy who brings brightness, compassion, a delicate masculine yet divinely feminine energy and sweet soul...and we would not be in as perfect a place without him.

I feel so blessed that I did not slip out of the system as so many women do. How many mothers and children have we seen perish all over the world for eons of time? I went through the private system and was able to be seen in a reasonably timely manner and was able to afford the help that I needed.

I worry what happens to those women with no financial capacity.

Women with no family support.

Women with an abusive partner.

Women who have to start work again immediately upon delivering.

Women who also have a sick child or chronically ill partner or older children.

What happens to these women who have PND and how are we not losing more women without the adequate support that they need? It also breaks my heart as to the *huge* impact that the current Covid restrictions and lockdowns are causing to our beautiful new families. If my family could not fly interstate to help me during that time, I truly am fearful as to what the outcome could have been. The additional fear, isolation and difficulties in accessing timely healthcare is a real and heavy additional weight that is the reality of the burden of this pandemic.

The additional birth trauma without support people allowed; the fear of contracting Covid whilst pregnant; the inability to join mother's groups for maternal support; or the inability of friends or family being able to come over and help in the way they normally could, are serious impediments to healing. I am currently in a lockdown in Sydney as I write this, so the tight restrictions on not being able to leave our local government area, border restrictions, not being able to leave home unless it is 'essential', and the pressures of job security and finances are real and all-consuming. The impact of this pandemic on the mental health of all people, let alone new mothers who may be suffering from post-natal depression, is one of grave concern and I truly hope that hospitals and obstetricians are watching closely and are providing additional support to our new mothers.

It does take a village to raise a child and I am grateful that I have and had mine. For those who are venturing on this journey alone, I would say, *please* do reach out to your family if you have them and are able to, or reach out to your friends and your community. Seek refuge wherever you feel comfortable and are able to access safely and are welcomed with an open heart and arms.

Now is the time to lean on whoever it is as your life-support and life-line.

Remove whatever feelings you may have that are holding you back and find support wherever it may lie for you. It is in times like these that you realise who is rallying behind you and who has your back. Ask your obstetrician, child health nurses, midwife or GP to help connect you with whatever services and support you need.

There is a world of support available if we just take one step towards accessing it.

May we not have to suffer alone any more, and may we continue to keep building and creating the best maternal mental healthcare facilities world-wide that do not feel so clinical and are completely focussed on the divine healing of our women.

That is my wish for the world moving forward.

HEALTH TIP:

It is important to discuss with your physician the possibility of any underlying health conditions that may be causing symptoms of anxiety and depression. It may be a good idea to get some baseline blood tests to ascertain certain biochemical markers and possible imbalances, that if restored may alleviate some of your physical symptoms. For example;

+ hypothyroidism (low thyroid) or hyperthyroidism (over active thyroid)

+ nutritional imbalances; such as iron or B6

+ alcohol and illicit drug use/misuse

+ adverse effects of certain medications (such as corticosteroids)

HEALTH TIP:

WHAT IS AVAILABLE FOR MOOD, ANXIETY AND SLEEP OVER THE COUNTER?

+ *It is important to discuss how you are feeling, what other medications and supplements that you are taking to your doctor or pharmacist before taking any over-the-counter medication. There can be drug interactions and considerations to be made about their safety, whether you are breastfeeding and whether there are alternatives available that are more suited for you*

+ *The following is not an exhaustive list and not intended to delve into clinical research as to their efficacy. They are available over-the-counter and should be discussed at length with your prescriber and pharmacist before starting or adding them onto any treatment regime.*

   - *Magnesium (powders, capsules, in bath soaks)*
   - *Vitamin B6 and the B-group vitamins in general during times of stress and requiring endurance*
   - *Bach Rescue Remedy- utilises homeopathy for calming the nervous system*
   - *Lavender and chamomile*
   - *St John's Wort (efficacy still requires extensive research, can interact with a lot of medications)*
   - *SAMe or 5HTP (precursor to serotonin)*
   - *Omega 3's*
   - *Melatonin (regulate the circadian rhythm for sleep)*
   - *Zizyphus (sleep)*
   - *Lemon Balm*
   - *Valerian (sleep)*
   - *Passionflower*
   - *Sedating anti-histamines on consultation with your pharmacist, yet these can interact with several medications and breastfeeding is a consideration to be made*

HEALTH TIP:

WHAT PRANAYAMAS/BREATHING TECHNIQUES ARE HELPFUL?
Pranayamas are breathing techniques that work in clearing the channels within the body as well as creating clarity, calm and focus within the mind. They can be used anywhere and allow your focus to return to your breath, which is very calming for anxiety symptoms as well as nervousness and fog in the head.

NADI SHODHANA OR ALTERNATE NOSTRIL BREATHING
Place your right thumb on your right nostril, your index and middle finger on your third eye point in between your eyebrows and your ring finger on your left nostril. Close your eyes and keep your thumb closing your right nostril as you breathe in through your left nostril, then exhale by closing your left nostril with your ring finger and breathing out through your right nostril. Then keeping your left nostril closed, breathe in through the right nostril and keep alternating breath like this as many times that feel good for you. It will bring clarity and oxygen into the mind and body.

BHASTRIKA OR BELLOWS BREATH - Not to be used if pregnant or on a full stomach. Sit with straight spine and stabilised core.

This is very uplifting and can enhance energy and improve focus if feeling sluggish. It requires a forceful inhalation and forceful exhalation from deep within the diaphragm and the nose. Forceful inhalation in with diaphragm pushing out and then forceful exhalation through the nose with the diaphragm pulling in towards the spine. Repeat as many times that feel good while creating an uplifting feeling within you.

HEALTH TIP:

WHAT SELF CARE STRATEGIES CAN I UTILISE?

+ _Go for a walk in nature_

+ _Have a herbal tea outside in the sun_

+ _Run a beautiful hot bath with a scented candle and some relaxing music_

+ _Dance if you love dancing_

+ _Read a book if you find that calming and relaxing_

+ _Call a friend or family member. Ask them to come over for a tea or coffee and talk_

+ _Bake if you enjoy baking or cooking_

+ _Exercise; yoga, do strength training, walk or run based on your ability_

+ _Have a shower, do a facial, give yourself a manicure or pedicure_

+ _Spend time cuddling your children and/or pet_

+ _Listen to music or your favourite podcast_

+ _Meditate; listening to music or a guided meditation if you cannot centre your thoughts_

+ _Take a nap_

+ _Get dressed up even if you have nowhere special to be; you will feel amazing_

+ _Journal in your favourite book with a cup of tea or nice yummy treat to eat_

CHAPTER 3

TAKE HOME MESSAGES

WHAT EXACTLY DID I FEEL WITHIN MYSELF WHEN I HAD POST-NATAL DEPRESSION?

- I felt completely crippled with anxiety which felt like hot knives stabbing me in the chest, pins and needles across my neck and down my arms 24/7

- I felt like my head was *constantly* in a thick dark black fog

- I could not make *any* decisions

- I would stare blankly into space and hours could pass by. I was completely unaware of the concept of time and my thoughts would run wild with anxiety or completely be lost in the black fog vortex

- I could not sleep at all. My anxiety would feel *crippling* and I would toss and turn ruminating through all of my incessant thoughts

- I would dread nights the most as there was only silence and nothing could steer me away from my crippling thoughts

- I had a dry mouth

- I could not smile

- I could not concentrate to watch T.V or a movie. I could not focus on anything at all

- I had zero appetite. I could not eat a morsel of food so ended up losing so much weight during those 11 weeks which would have caused me to go into starvation mode and wreaked havoc on my metabolism

- I would constantly go over my repetitive loop to anyone around me

- I could not have any coherent conversations about anything other than that dreaded loop

- I felt *empty* inside. No emotion at all

- I felt so alone and *scared*. I felt *utterly* hopeless and crippled with fear

- I felt like there was no way out and I had no idea what would change this or how long this would go on for

- I had suicidal ideations and would imagine *all* the different ways to make this all disappear. This was the scariest part of all. Frightening. It would *haunt* me

- My repetitive loop at least stopped me from my ideations but when there was no one listening to me, my ideations would take hold

- Every moment felt torturous. I felt *trapped* inside my body but I didn't feel like me. At all. I knew that I had vanished and it felt so frustrating

- I could not do simple tasks; picking an outfit, expressing milk felt too complicated, it took 45 minutes to make a formula bottle, basic self-care was neglected unless I had a doctor's appointment, but it would take every ounce of energy to pull myself together to get there. Then I fell into a heap at the end of it all. I simply could not function at all

- I wanted to bury my head under my blankets especially in the morning when I would hear the kids wake up. I wished that I could be swallowed up whole, so would hide in bed even though I had not and could not sleep. I just remained in a foetal position in my bed for hours at a time

- I had no initiative or motivation to do anything. I couldn't make decisions, so even to go for a walk someone would have to instigate and take the lead of taking me with them otherwise I would not go outside

- I would sit alone in my room for *hours* ruminating in silence

- I would do basic things with the baby or Ari but my heart was not connected. Conversation felt forced and unnatural and I just went through the motions, not really engaging in any of it

- I wanted someone to magically fix it, but felt *so stuck.* Stuck in mud and suffocated by every aspect of it

WHAT DID I STRUGGLE WITH THE MOST?

1. I struggled with going from a fully functioning Type A personality who rules the home with how it operates and making decisions; to becoming a person who could not make decisions, could not think and became so dependent upon everyone to do everything. This transpired literally overnight. That was *truly* difficult. It also added to the feelings of guilt and shame, that I

felt like I was burdening everyone and like I was failing my duty as a mother.

2. I struggled with the physical symptoms as well as not being able to do anything. I was in my physical body but not really there at all.

3. I struggled with not being able to have a conversation. It sounds ludicrous now but I truly could not talk at all unless it was about my loop.

4. I struggled with not remembering or knowing how I interacted or connected with Ari and Ruphus. I didn't know what we did together or what we would talk about. They knew this too, so didn't want to be around me. I had left my body and I was not there anymore. That was hard too because I wanted to be around them but I just didn't know how to be other than silent, so I felt even more alone and empty.

WHAT MADE MY JOURNEY OF RECOVERY EASIER?

1. The fact that everyone around me was helping and taking on so much more than they needed to, just so I could focus on healing and recovering. My husband took on so many extra duties and roles without any sleep on top of keeping the bills, businesses and our life ticking over as before. My parents and in-laws kept our household going with *everything* that is involved with that whilst they were living with us from interstate; without which we could *not* have survived at all. My brother and sister would call and message multiple times throughout the day to check in on how I was going. I never felt like I was going through this alone.

2. *Everyone* in our family put their own lives aside. They all had their own jobs, children, businesses or work that they still had to do but they *all* created time in their days to support us 100 percent. They invested so much time and effort in me. That requires so much patience and selflessness and I will be forever grateful for all of them in creating room in their time for me. The toll that it would have placed on their shoulders and lives is not unnoticed and is so *sincerely* appreciated and acknowledged.

3. Without all of their help we would have sunk. *All* of us. There would have been no way that the pressure of the severity of my illness would not have crumbled Chandi to the ground and these poor children would be completely alone.

4. Our family carried us through this chapter. Without a doubt and without them, we would not be here living such a wonderful life. We can say thank you but nothing will ever articulate or repay what each and every one of them gave to us during the hardest time of our lives.

If you have family, please lean on them. Use them as your life raft.

If you don't, then call on your friends and remove any guilt or feelings of embarrassment or shame and just reach out.

If you don't have family *or* friends, then reach out to someone in your community; your neighbour, someone from the school or local café. Who knows what support they may be willing to give you. Do not feel like you need to conquer this alone. It will make the path harder and rockier without having a tribe to help you along this journey. If all else fails, ring 000 to be taken to where there is professional help or discuss support options with your GP or obstetrician.

If you are reading this and know someone who has had a baby, then use it as an opportunity to ask them how they are doing. Create space for them to let you know that they may need some help and allow yourself to be a vehicle of service for this family. They will hold you in their hearts forever and the support that you give them could well be an actual life line.

WHAT MADE MY JOURNEY HARDER?

1. Not knowing exactly when I would recover was the hardest part for all of us, because we never knew how long the darkness would shadow our lives. It becomes difficult to hold onto faith and hold on when the end point is not known. I know we do not have a crystal ball but that was the *hardest* part.

2. The added strains within relationship dynamics from this stressful situation, created more heaviness in my heart and shoulders. I would say that if any interaction does not have the patient at the forefront and focus, then it is having the opposite impact that is required.

   Do not allow extra pressures that are not necessary to weigh more heavily on the patient, as her *sole* function and focus needs to be on her recovery. Nothing more and nothing less.

3. I also found it difficult having children in different States and not having them in Sydney where I grew up. I was in a situation each time of not knowing what help was available and where I needed to go or who to see. I was not aware of the services available in Cairns with Ari or Perth with Kaiyaan, so I truly felt lost and overwhelmed. Without the cognition to actively look as I normally would have, I, as the patient, could not do that alone. I needed someone to take the reins and take charge of my medical emergency to find someone to see.

I would say that if you are recognising that you may require help and cannot take the reins to find someone, then reach out to your partner, family or friends and ask them to take charge of this for you. The sooner you speak to someone and start your treatment journey, whatever that may be, the sooner you can put all of this behind you.

Ask them to take charge.

Let them take charge.

If you are a family member or partner reading this and are recognising similarities in my symptoms and presentation, then it is *your* duty to take charge and get them in to see someone ASAP. No one realises how serious this can be until sometimes it is *too* late. We cannot afford to lose one more soul to this.

Look out for the signs. Do not wait for time to make it better as chances are that it may remain the same or get worse. Far worse.

Remember the pressure, strain and stress of the current situation can only linger by no one taking action. Create space and action towards finding who you need to see and walk yourself or allow someone to help carry you to the other side.

I promise you the sweetness that lies on the other side is *so* divine. It *is* there, I promise.

It is like honey and it will taste even sweeter when you get there.

> *HEALTH TIP:*
>
> *WHAT ARE THE BENEFITS OF INFANT MASSAGE? Ref: Infant Massage Information Service (IMIS)*
>
> *+ It can enhance bonding and attachment for both mother and baby*
>
> *+ It can increase the neurotransmitters Serotonin and Dopamine for both mother and baby; which can enhance mood, reduce anxiety and can help sleep*
>
> *+ It can increase Oxytocin, the 'love hormone' for both mother and baby*
>
> *+ It can reduce Cortisol, the stress hormone for both mother and baby*
>
> *+ It can strengthen the immune system of the baby and reduce crying*
>
> *+ It can increase weight gain for low birth weight babies*
>
> *+ It can act as a pain reliever by enhancing endorphins which can be helpful for colic, teething and wind*
>
> *+ It can enhance the vagal nerve activity, which is the biggest nerve in the gut-brain axis. This can positively affect the digestive, respiratory and circulatory systems*
>
> *+ It can enhance the confidence and self-esteem for the mother that they are able to provide comfort*

PART 2

SUPPORT TOOLS

The purpose of part 2 is so that if you are going through post-natal depression yourself and are finding that reading my story in the earlier parts is triggering or it simply contains *too* much information to read; I totally get it! Skip straight to this part so that you can read my point by point thoughts about:

- Post-natal depression facts broken down
- Reflections and take home messages
- Views on mindset
- Implications of self-talk
- Information about the hormonal shift that occurs post-birth
- Thoughts and stance on medication and treatments
- Practical support tools for the mother
- Practical support tools for the spouse, children and parents/families
- Healing exercises
- Resources for support access

I would like to acknowledge that being this raw and vulnerable by picking apart my experience and learnings was *not* an easy task, as I am expressing such profound and very sad thoughts that I was having at the time. I love my boys with every cell of my being so reliving this experience again has been quite confronting.

However, I have held *all* of you women that are suffering through this deep within my heart. Hopefully you gain some insight and respite into how you are feeling and so that you do not need to feel trapped in the position you are currently in. I hope that the points can provide you with some solace and peace of mind but most importantly, I hope that it can give you achievable strategies to step forward into your recovery, as well as so much *hope.*

I initiated an experiment from pregnancy A to pregnancy B by changing *every* single variable between them and had the *exact* same outcome (except the use of an epidural in both births and the use of Motilium (Domperidone) to enhance milk supply with my second baby). This has allowed for me to know deep within my heart that we *cannot* control suffering from post-natal depression, and that the way we give birth or navigate through pregnancy do not 'cause' post-natal depression per se.

Pregnancy A I gained A LOT of weight. I stopped working at 6 months, I was not very active, I was not mindful of optimal foetal positioning and ended up having an emergency C-section. I had trouble with my milk supply as well as latching and breastfeeding. My parents were far away until week three and I did not have a tribe around me, being a first-time Mum in a new place where I hadn't lived before.

Pregnancy B I gained around one third of the amount of weight. I worked right up until 38-weeks and I did Hypnobirthing to prepare for a VBAC which I was successful in achieving. I did antenatal yoga weekly, I focused on optimal foetal positioning, joined the ABA (Australian Breastfeeding Association) during pregnancy to make sure that I had contacts and help available from the outset with breastfeeding. I had acupuncture weekly for my fluid retention and then preparation for labour closer to delivery and had Reiki once a month for the entire pregnancy. My parents flew in to Perth at 38 weeks gestation and we had family support around us for a full 3 months. I felt like I had the polar opposite variables, hoping that it would lead to a different outcome.

However, despite the 180-degree difference in pregnancies, not only was my second post-natal depression *far* worse, but exactly on day 5 for both boys, like clock-work my body flicked the switch on to the deepest, darkest and most harrowing post-natal depression. At exactly 11 weeks post-birth each time and taking different medications starting at different times, my body re-emerged back into my true self and the dark cloud encompassing my whole being lifted and went back to wherever it came from.

It swiftly lasted for this entire duration of my 'fourth trimester' of pregnancy. Whilst swiftly it came and went, it managed to leave a trail of trauma and pain that required a lot of healing throughout that time. Swift it may have been, yet it ravaged through all aspects of my life and home and the darkness clutched its claws into everyone closest to me.

The pain was real and dark.

The effects of the hormonal influence on the biochemistry of my brain were so profound and marked, that arguably even without any pre-existing anxiety or depression, it had the capacity to completely destroy a perfectly healthy body and mind. It left a lasting imprint on the hearts, minds and souls of all those involved.

My biggest struggle was in not knowing how long I would have post-natal depression for, which made holding and hanging on so much more difficult each and every day. I did not know when the light at the end of the tunnel would present. I did not even know or at times even believe, that there *was* a light there waiting for me.

Especially the first time.

This unknowing, tests the release of the 'control' element so profoundly because one has to hold onto faith in something or someone that is far greater than our self. This in itself can be so challenging and tests the strength in everyone involved in holding on, in the hope of a better and brighter road ahead.

Unlike a physical surgery where a clear map can be carved out with regard to your healing, post-natal depression does not have a one size fits all approach. Everyone may have different presenting symptoms or severity of illness. However, speaking up about how you are feeling less than optimal IS the most important piece of the puzzle to move towards your healing.

Whilst no doctor or psychologist can give you a definite date of return, we can all unequivocally say that you *will* get better. It may take going through one treatment tool at a time, adding more as you realise what is helping and what is not. Time for each medication to work is also necessary to allow for them to take hold, which means that it can be an exercise of patience to find the right key for your lock.

There will be resistant, stubborn and very difficult cases without a doubt, yet I do truly believe that with ongoing support and treatment that eventually *even* these cases will find some respite. It is always so vital to keep on holding on and to *never ever* give up.

You deserve to feel better. You have earned it.

I hope that you can find peace in your heart and mind in trusting that you *will* get through this time. Though you may not feel like this is possible right now, I *promise* you that with time, success is achievable.

I found that when I was going through it, that whilst there was information explaining what PND is and resources present to seek help, I didn't know if what I was feeling was 'normal'. I also did not have access to tools to help nourish my recovery at home whilst I was either waiting to get into medical treatment or whilst waiting for medication to work...I was literally waiting silently in my closed room for a magical shift to happen, which made my days so painful for myself and my entire family.

The stress of going to different appointments when I had no cognitive function, could not make decisions and complete simple tasks, seemed almost impossible. This all added up to make the whole process very stressful and painful. If I wasn't on the phone or going to appointments, I would lock myself in our room like a leper or hermit with my repetitive loop, and not do anything to help focus my attention *away* from the reality of the pain that was.

Not because I didn't want to, but because I didn't have the *ability* to take the reins towards action and do the things that I knew would help me.

What I needed were tools to subconsciously initiate healing and respite instead of sitting in a silent room *waiting* for a miraculous event to bring that healing to me. I believe that subtle and additive effects from various modalities would have supported and nourished my body, mind and nervous system, that may have allowed for a faster recovery or at least create subtle healing and respite in the background *whilst* accessing Western healthcare at the same time. This is the purpose of creating this tool and all of the others, to give you practical and accessible tools to help you on your journey of healing...No longer do I want other mothers to think '*I feel this way, now what?*'

I also want to break the stigma of speaking out and accessing and seeking medical treatments, whether it be medication and/or cognitive behavioural therapy and all the other type of treatments in between that are available. There is no shame or danger in accessing such treatments, and they did in fact SAVE MY LIFE without a shadow of a doubt. Twice.

For those against medication, I implicitly want to explain that it is not addictive, nor a Band-Aid solution. Rather, it is a way to help repair and rebalance a biochemical imbalance, that once restored can allow for you to step into the optimum level of thriving for your body; IF that is what your healing needs and your medical team deem is appropriate. They can be weaned down after your recovery with the guidance of your prescriber and you do not have to remain on them forever, as some people may believe.

I also understand that there are side effects associated with medication and that is a reality of the duality of pharmaceuticals. What can be life transforming can also cause other unwanted effects; sometimes mild, transient and other times more profound. These can be discussed with your prescriber and with open communication and information, it hopefully allows for transparency in your decision-making process. As a pharmacist I can *fully* appreciate and acknowledge this aspect of medications and hope that I can educate where needed in this regard.

Getting psychotherapy allows you to view and modify your mindsets, work through certain triggers and layers that may be sources of trauma, or self-talk that may be affecting the way you view life. It can help to change the filter or lens through which you view life and once completed you will re-emerge as the strongest, most dynamic, lightest, more aligned and grounded in your true values and most authentic self you could possibly ever dream of becoming.

Despite undertaking a lot of reflection and healing, we as a family at times still need to heal aspects that re-present throughout our lives together. We had nowhere to go but to heal, shed the outdated belief systems, layers of values that no longer served us and to step into constantly evolving, whilst living with so much gratitude to have health and breath in our body.

Whilst you are in a dark space I can FULLY appreciate that this may feel like a lot of work. Yet, I want to say to hold on and keep strong in the knowing that healing IS possible. Healing can and will come, and though our journeys are all different and filled with so many variables, I do understand that there are 'no one size fits all' solutions. However, you must keep taking steps forward one breath at a time towards your goal. It is also important to say that it is a process of patience, as unlike other things in life where there is a very quick cause and effect process, this sometimes can be a longer process...but that should encourage you to speak up as soon as you can, so that you are going to be closer to feeling better sooner, than letting the situation linger.

If you as a mother are finding it difficult to focus your attention on reading, which I will admit I would have found almost impossible; then I would suggest your partner, spouse, family member or friend read this and gain helpful tools, so that they can guide you in utilising steps towards your road to recovery.

I hope that everyone in the world who knows someone having or who has had a baby can read this, and start the conversation as to how to be of service to a new mother. This hopefully can make your journey to recovery and back to your light easier, less stressful and less isolating than necessary.

Life at home after having a baby does not always look picture perfect and it is time to break the illusion of that, so that you can find strength in being vulnerable and authentic in your situation.

This 'picture perfect' ideology for those with PND seems like a destination so far from their reality, that it makes it feel like recovery is impossible or that the road is too long and hard to travel.

Yet, if you start with even one tool, one piece of support advice or healing modality listed, hopefully it adds nourishment and enrichment into your healing journey. Incorporate as many as you can achieve comfortably *without* feeling overwhelmed.

Sign up to a meal train, say yes when friends offer to bring you food, subscribe to a food service, download the sound healings or other e-books or whatever it is that you are drawn towards to make your road less rocky.

Support people who are encouraging of these insights and healing modalities and take charge in allowing it to occur, will definitely make the mother feel supported, seen and heard. She will feel held in a way that will embrace her body, mind and soul and allow for a truly connected experience together, aligned with the same goal for her recovery.

By taking one step in front of the other you are showing commitment and a dedication towards your children, your partner and yourself that you are willing to do whatever it takes to receive the healing that your body needs. Allow it. Accept it. Embrace it.

Remember that you are deserving and seeking help and support is *not* selfish but a sign of self-respect and self-love. You are worthy and you deserve to be connected to your light again and the world is supporting you to return back to your light because we need you. All of you. Right now x

HEALTH TIP:

THE GUT-BRAIN AXIS CONNECTION

+ _There is consistently more research into the Gut-Brain connection, indicating that the gut microbiome and gut-health is interlinked with neurotransmitter production affecting moods and hormones within the body_

+ _The vagus nerve is one of the biggest nerves that connects the gut to the brain. Interestingly infant massage positively impacts the vagus nerve, thereby enhancing digestion, circulation and respiration in the baby_

+ _The gut microbiome produces GABA which is the inhibitory neurotransmitter, that controls fear and anxiety. Interestingly my blood results showed low GABA and I have struggled with my gut health for some time_

+ _Some studies have illustrated that certain probiotics have the ability to increase GABA production, which therefore would reduce symptoms of anxiety which illustrates this gut-brain connection further_

+ _Inflammation has also been found to exist in a number of brain disorders. Dr Serrallach's book The Postnatal Depletion Cure discusses the presence of inflammatory neuropeptides as being one of the reasons for causing neurological symptoms post-delivery_

+ _The gut plays a vital role in our immune system and inflammatory response, so good gut health is crucial for overall health and well-being_

+ _The digestive fire strength or agni in Ayurveda, is considered the most fundamental cornerstone in one's health and forms the basis of all disease processes. A strong digestive fire has the ability for the body to digest and assimilate nutrients from food, whereas a weakened digestive fire has the capacity to create undigested material called Ama, that can accumulate within the system and begin the disease process_

What can help restore or maintain a healthy gut?

+ _Firstly, it is vital to see your physician and rule out any underlying health conditions, intolerances and to review your medications, especially regular use of antibiotics_

+ _Other things that potentially may have an impact on the quality of your gut health include;_

- Probiotics and Prebiotics

- Digestive enzymes

- Fish oil which contain omega 3's and EPA and DHA as anti-inflammatory agents

- Fermented foods and foods that reduce inflammation within the body (gluten and casein-protein for example, can be quite inflammatory)

- High fibre foods; care with any intolerances that you may exhibit. Seeing an APD (Accredited Practising Dietician can help navigate your way through nutrition and specific dietary advice)

- Polyphenol rich foods (berries, cocoa, flaxseeds and olives as some examples)

- Tryptophan rich foods (turkey, chicken, oatmeal, nuts, eggs, tofu as some examples)

- Ginger and black pepper are excellent spices in Ayurveda that can stimulate the digestive fire

- Avoiding cold or icy drinks, especially at meal times as well as not drinking too much water within 30 minutes of meal times, as they can dampen the digestive fire or agni in Ayurveda

CHAPTER 1

POST-NATAL DEPRESSION BROKEN DOWN

WHAT IS POST-NATAL DEPRESSION?

This is a very serious and debilitating condition that is associated with negative emotional changes that last for 2 weeks or longer after having a baby. It is generally accepted to occur within the first 12-months after delivery.

For some women it can happen immediately and a drastic change seen overnight; as was the case for me.

For some women, symptoms may slowly present or appear after a few months.

WHAT ARE THE SYMPTOMS?

Symptoms can range from presenting with some or all of the manifestations listed below, and can occur to varying degrees between all women. There is not necessarily a 'one size fits all' presentation of PND, suffice to say that all women would feel *less* than their optimal and thriving self.

Some women may be able to observe and identify these within themselves, or may require their partner, family or friend to identify signs and symptoms, in order to assist in taking the next step of diagnosis and treatment.

- *Inability to concentrate or make decisions*
- *Anger or frustration*
- *Feeling no emotion or low and numb*
- *Feeling teary or sad all the time*
- *Lack of interest or pleasure in things normally enjoyable; even time with your baby*
- *No motivation, no energy*
- *Changes in sleep; sleeping too much or not able to sleep at all*
- *Changes in eating; eating more or less than usual*
- *No hope for the future*
- *Feeling like you are unable to cope and things are too overwhelming*
- *Feeling very teary or emotional*
- *Feeling isolated, alone and disconnected from others*
- *Having thoughts of self-harming or harming your baby*
- *Anxiety*
- *Heavy and clouded feeling in the head; cannot think clearly*
- *Losing confidence*
- *Fears of being alone or fear of being around people*
- *Feeling like your baby does not love you or that you don't love your baby*
- *Inability to do regular everyday tasks*
- *Disconnection from your baby and children; lack of connection and emotion*
- *Inability to function which makes everything feel difficult and overwhelming*
- *Feeling like there is no way out, stuck, no hope or nothing will get you out*
- *Loss of joy, emotion and pleasure in things you normally love*

WHAT ARE PRE-DISPOSING FACTORS FOR HAVING POST-NATAL DEPRESSION?

There are some factors that may pre-dispose someone to having post-natal depression and include, but are not limited to, the following;

1. Family history or personal history of anxiety or depression
2. Birth disappointment
3. Traumatic birth; akin to PTSD
4. Relationship difficulties within the home
5. Fertility issues or previous loss of pregnancy
6. Controlling or abusive behaviour in a partner and/or family violence
7. Underlying medical condition; e.g. thyroid dysfunction, iron levels, low vitamin B6
8. Other medication that you are taking
9. Stressful life events
10. A difficult pregnancy
11. Lack of social support or isolation
12. Financial difficulties
13. Past history of abuse
14. History of severe PMS

HOW IS PND DIAGNOSED?

If you have any or all of the symptoms listed above for a period of 2 WEEKS OR MORE, then this can be a helpful guide as to whether you need to speak with your GP, obstetrician, midwife or child health nurse.

The 'Baby Blues' is having similar symptoms that can arrive at the onset of milk supply production around day 3 to day 5, but the time duration is short-lived compared to PND. This is a key differentiating factor that can help initiate a diagnosis and treatment plan to move forward.

The support team of your GP, obstetrician, midwife or child health nurse may give you a screening tool called the *EPDS, or the Edinburgh Postnatal Depression Scale*. This is not a diagnostic tool per se, but is a helpful screening tool to gauge how you are feeling in a measurable and quantifiable way. This can be useful considering that the symptoms can be hard to quantify without a scale or if you are having trouble articulating exactly what you are feeling.

I would encourage you to visit the COPE website (Centre of Perinatal Excellence) that has the full *EPDS* resource there and a lot of pertinent information about it. If you do feel like you may have PND then ask your provider to give you the *EPDS* if they have not done so already. Remove any fear of judgement when completing the form and be entirely *honest* with *how* you are feeling.

Whilst I have not included a copy of the *EPDS* here, however as a guide, the questions that are included on the tool have a range of answer scales and marking as to how you have felt in the *previous 7 days* and are listed below for your reference:

1. I have been able to laugh and see the funny side of things
2. I have looked forward with enjoyment to things
3. I have blamed myself unnecessarily when things have gone wrong
4. I have been anxious or worried for no good reason
5. I have felt scared or panicky for no good reason
6. Things have been getting on top of me
7. I have been so unhappy that I have had difficulty sleeping
8. I have felt sad or miserable
9. I have been so unhappy that I have been crying
10. The thought of harming myself has occurred to me

I remember I was scared to do this test as I was *petrified* of getting in trouble or that they would take my children or myself away. This was catastrophic thinking and held me back for so many weeks the first time in accessing the help that I needed, which was a monumental waste of time on reflection!

Doctors can also rule out other underlying conditions that may be causing your anxiety and depression symptoms by doing blood tests or using other differential diagnostic tools. They can review your medications and past medical history and make a diagnosis from all of this information provided to them. We are so blessed here in Australia to have access to high quality healthcare and *this* would be the time to access it and utilise it to your advantage.

This is the *first* step in accessing the tailor-made treatment for you, so please do not be afraid! Go to the doctor with your partner or family member to fill you with the confidence to be honest, and to not feel alone. If you feel like you would be more honest and transparent with your health provider if you went alone, then leave the baby with your partner or family.

Write a list of points and questions before going so that you feel properly armed in making the most out of the appointment. Ask for a long appointment time so you don't feel rushed and then you can relax more to better describe how you're feeling. Then you can more easily ascertain the best course of action for your unique circumstances.

The first step *can* and *did* feel so daunting for me and like a mammoth task! Working as a pharmacist, I would refer all of my patients to a doctor, yet when it came to *my* time I was riddled with fear...but let it go! If you cannot call to arrange an appointment, then partners/carers can step in to take *this* step for you! The sooner you all take the first step in seeking treatment, the sooner you can move away from the darkness and back into your life.

I would also say that upon acknowledging that you are ready to seek treatment, I encourage you to write a statement of commitment to yourself that you are prepared to do whatever it takes, to step into your healing. Write a statement of **your 'why'** and place it somewhere to constantly remind you of what you have committed to and why.

This will keep you motivated and accountable in *never* giving up, as you have made a promise and pledge to yourself and your loved ones of moving towards your recovery.

It will empower and motivate you profoundly.

WHERE DO I GO FOR HELP?

1. Call your obstetrician, GP, midwife or child health nurse depending on who you feel most comfortable with. They may all be in contact with each other and can collaborate with taking charge of your care.

   If you are unsure where to start, then your GP may be the best place to start. They can chat with your obstetrician on your behalf and act as triage in directing you where you need to go in a timely and effective manner. They can arrange referrals to wherever they feel most appropriate for you.

2. Ask for a long appointment upon booking and your GP can write a Mental Health Plan, which will create a specific plan of whom you need to see and you can access (currently) 20 bulk-billed sessions through Medicare to a psychologist per calendar year; though this number may change once Covid has passed.

   They can also write a referral within this plan to a psychiatrist who can manage your treatment options. If you have specific providers that you know you want to attend, then your GP can facilitate this for you. Discuss your financial capacity with them also, as different providers have different fee structures that may affect your out-of-pocket costs. Affordable health care will allow longevity and completion of treatment, which is the optimum outcome here for everyone!

3. There is a list of other lifeline support resources on the back pages of this book in Chapter 10, if you need to speak to someone urgently or whilst this is all unfolding. Organisations such as Lifeline, PANDA, Beyond Blue, the Gidget Foundation are some examples here in Australia, so do take a look and access anyone that you feel may help you.

4. Ideally your GP will refer you to a specific psychologist, otherwise ask for them to refer you to a perinatal-specific psychologist and psychiatrist that are well versed in post-natal depression, as this will make their help specific to your situation. Access APS (Australian Psychological Society) to search for specific psychologists or yourhealthinmind.org if you want to search for a psychiatrist yourself prior to the appointment. I found seeing The Elizabeth Clinic in Perth, which was a perinatal-specific practice, absolutely perfect for me as my doctor knew *exactly* what was happening with me and took charge with absolute confidence and skill, which took away any doubt or concern within me and I felt so held and seen in this framework.

5. Discuss with your GP about any additional support services that may benefit you to gain the *maximum* amount of support; social workers, child health nurses, lactation consultants, women's health physios, birth trauma counsellors etc. Ask what support services are available near you and get them to arrange everything they can, as easily as possible for you. There is so much help at hand if you ask for it and set any fear aside...as fear will hold you back.

You don't know what you don't know, and you cannot find out what help is available without saying that you need it! We are truly blessed in Australia in the care that is available, so speak up and see what can be arranged for you.

WHAT TREATMENTS ARE AVAILABLE?

It is not my place here to go through every medication or treatment option, as it will depend on your individual symptoms and your doctor. However, to allay any doubt in your mind that effective treatment *is* available in changing this biochemical imbalance, and how you are feeling, this is what I will stress here!

I thought that there was nothing that anyone could do, say or give me that would change my problem, which was regretting having a baby in amongst my anxiety, insomnia and depression! Those feelings *only* existed because of my imbalance and literally disappeared the moment my medication worked and the imbalance was corrected! Imagine if I hadn't taken action and was forced to continue living such a disconnected and depressed life forever!

I shudder at the thought, because treatment *was* what allowed me to *feel* different and the effects were undeniable, and came as abruptly/quickly as my symptoms had set in. It truly was magic. I also shudder at the thought of the time when medication was not available, or for people who cannot access medication or treatment. There would be no way that lives would not be lost to this condition. Science is magic; truly.

Treatment does and can work for you too...I promise! Not all agents work effectively or the same way for every person, but your health triage team can work through option by option until you all get the desired outcome. Do not think that because a certain treatment worked for a friend or another mother that it will work for you or vice versa. There is a lock and key for each of us that has its own unique combination that needs to be worked out.

Options that your GP, psychologist or psychiatrist can choose from, include but are not limited to;

1. MEDICATIONS

   - To help *insomnia* symptoms (range of options that work in different ways)
   - To help *anxiety* symptoms (range of options)
   - To help lift the *depression* symptoms (range of options to use that work in different ways)

   You may need one, or a combination of a few different types, depending on your symptoms and presentation. Trust your team and trust in the process.

   Not every medication will work the same way in every person and the same medication may have worked once, but may not work the second time. It is the nature of the beast.

   For antidepressants it may take 1 to 3 weeks to see some positive effect. It may take 4 to 6 weeks to see most of the effects occur and may take 6 to 8 weeks for the *full* effects to take place.

   Watch, observe and allow your family to be the sounding board to give feedback on how well it is helping with your symptoms and *be patient!*

2. PSYCHOTHERAPY

   This can be CBT (Cognitive Behavioural Therapy), IPT (Interpersonal Therapy), Behaviour Therapy, MBCT (Mindfulness-Based Cognitive Therapy) or counselling. There are a variety of tools that psychologists and psychiatrists can utilise, depending on exactly what you require. Their knowledge in this field is exemplary and you will be amazed at how they can offer you the exact tools and coping strategies, amongst other things to help navigate you through this illness and any feelings surrounding birth trauma or anything else you need.

3. ECT - ELECTROCONVULSIVE THERAPY

This is another tool that can be utilised by a psychiatrist, if they deem necessary and appropriate.

WHAT CAN I DO FOR MY ANXIETY SYMPTOMS?

If you are feeling anxious, then the first thing is to speak with your GP and include this information for them to tailor make your Mental Health Plan, as well as discussing practical tools from your psychologist and/or psychiatrist.

However, things that *can* help with anxiety symptoms include the following strategies;

- deep breathing
- meditation; guided meditation for an overactive mind
- counting to ten whilst breathing deeply as a mindful and focussed tool
- focus on the things around the room, with full presence and do not let the anxious thoughts overpower your taking in the aspects of the room
- journaling through any underlying reason or trigger causing it
- exercise and yoga
- reduce caffeine
- reduce alcohol and avoid illicit drugs

- prana (life-force) rich nutrition; fresh produce, home-cooked with less processed/fast food or convenient packaged type food
- identify any triggers that can worsen it; e.g. skipping a meal, certain food or news channels
- identify any activities that help *you* get through the anxious feelings

In terms of supplements, I would encourage you to seek all treatment through your prescriber from the outset. Now that you are accessing help, this is not the time to experiment with over-the-counter options, unless your doctor has recommended them for you and would have seen first-hand what effects they can exert on their patients. Whilst natural supplements exist naturally in the environment, it does not mean that every single one is effective, nor does it mean that there may not be some side effects and interactions with other medications and specific medical conditions. They can have drug interactions with what your prescriber has given, so full transparency with your health team is encouraged here, for your safety and optimum health outcome.

However, supplement options for anxiety *can* include the following list; though I have not entered into the scientific or clinical research data of the efficacy of each listed agent. It is more a list of strategies that are available to access, however please do speak with your triage team as to what exactly is recommended for you.

1. Prescription medication options are available for short-term use if very severe, or for short-term situations such as PND
2. Magnesium can assist as a muscle relaxant and calming agent
3. Chamomile
4. B-group vitamins; especially B-Complex

5. Vitamin D if it is low in your system, which is becoming increasingly more common
6. Bach Rescue Remedy (homeopathic preparation that may assist with anxiety)
7. Earthy and grounding scents like frankincense, lavender, myrrh, neroli
8. Omega-3 fatty acid supplements
9. Lemon Balm
10. Valerian
11. GABA; the inhibitory neurotransmitter associated with anxiety
12. Probiotic and assessing gut-health

WHAT CAN I DO IF I HAVE A PANIC ATTACK?

When you have post-natal depression, PNDA or anxiety, there can be times when you may feel like you are having or are actually having a panic attack.

A panic attack can come on suddenly through a trigger, through excessive stimuli or it may present out of nowhere in the most unlikely scenarios. It can appear with any of the following symptoms;

- Nausea, or abdominal pain/discomfort
- Chills or hot flushes
- Sweating
- Dry mouth
- Trembling or shaking
- Numbness or tingling of the chest, hands or legs
- Dizziness
- Heart palpitations or an increased pounding of the heart; some people worry that it is a heart attack
- Hyperventilation; shallow and fast breaths

- Feeling like the walls are closing in around you; feeling of suffocating

If this happens to you, then try to utilise some of these strategies to get you through the attack. Then call your doctor and triage team of psychologist and/or psychiatrist so you can talk this through in case it happens again, and they can give specific strategies for you:

- Close your eyes and block out all of the unnecessary stimuli

- Focus on your breathing; and make DEEP, CONTROLLED, FOCUSSED BREATHS... concentrate on the DEEP BREATH IN and HOLD...then EXHALE SLOWLY. It may help to count to 5 with each SLOW inhalation and count to 5 with each SLOW exhalation. Not only will the slow breathing calm the sympathetic nervous system, it can help to take focus away from the panic

- If you prefer to focus on a particular object if you feel too scared to close your eyes...then gaze and bring your awareness to an object and try to block out everything else

- Tell yourself 'THIS WILL PASS'...or 'RIDE THE WAVE', repeat a favourite and relaxing mantra or focus word like 'RELAX, FOCUS'...whatever resonates with you and allows you to come back into your body

- If you find it helpful to call a friend or family member during the attack and are able to; then call them and let them talk you through it. Having that support can feel like a beautiful shoulder to lean on and they will be so happy to be there for you when you need it the most

- If you can go for a walk or do some gentle exercise to focus your attention elsewhere; such as on the beautiful nature around you, the pavement or the sky, then move your body through the physical symptoms and this can be extremely helpful for some

- If you have lavender, frankincense or a calming scent that you connect with then, allow your senses to focus on the smell as this can be very calming and grounding

If your partner is having a panic attack, then be there to support and reassure them that they will get through this;

- Stay calm within yourself

- Name it; say 'you are having a panic attack but you *will* get through this'

- Be encouraging and supportive without judgement or annoyance

- If they have had it before and you know what helps, then utilise those strategies

- Tell them coping statements to reassure them; 'This will pass', 'You can get through this', 'Breathe in and hold for 5, then breathe out for the count of 5'

- If they like touch, then gently place your hand on their back; otherwise if they do not, just be there for them and reassure them and let them know that you are by their side the entire time

- Always use a slow and comforting tone of voice

It can be very energetically draining after having a panic attack so allow them to rest, make sure they remain hydrated, have a nourishing meal and simply be there for them and allay any fears surrounding it. Contact her healthcare team and establish a game plan moving forward, so that you all feel better equipped should it happen again.

WHAT CAN I DO FOR MY DEPRESSION SYMPTOMS?

The best thing you can do is to be honest with how you feel to your doctor so that they can assess the best course of treatment for you. There are many classes of pharmacological agents that can help to bring balance to biochemistry, depending on your specific presenting symptoms. Therapeutic Guidelines have medically accepted treatment protocols and it will be up to your prescriber as to what they feel is best for you.

However, in addition to Western medication, other lifestyle strategies that *may* assist in synergy can include;

1. Exercise; even as little as 20-minutes per day can enhance endorphins and 'good chemicals'
2. Eat nutritionally dense food and Prana (life-force) rich food vs packaged and 'convenient' type foods that are processed and refined that are devoid of nutrients
3. Try to eat on time and not skip meals
4. Try to sleep in the closest type of routine as possible
5. Reduce stress
6. Reduce alcohol and illicit drugs
7. Mindfulness practices; yoga, breathing, meditation
8. Self-care strategies
9. Connecting with family and friends
10. Omega supplements, probiotics for gut health, B-group vitamins
11. Reviewing blood work to find any underlying deficiency; zinc, thyroid function, iron, B-group vitamins as some basic examples

12. Whilst there are natural supplements that are anecdotally used for symptoms of depression, for example St John's Wort is very common, but they can interact with *various* medications and supplements, so require full disclosure before commencing or adding this into your treatment without medical supervision

WHAT CAN I DO FOR MY INSOMNIA?

Speak to your GP, psychologist and psychiatrist about your symptoms to best tailor your treatment according to how you are feeling. They can ascertain what is best for *you* as there are various classes of medication that work in different ways pharmacologically speaking.

However, the following are some sleep hygiene strategies that are also listed elsewhere in the book, and may give you an outline as to what strategies may promote and encourage sleep, which I believe is a vital step in the healing and rejuvenation process post-birth;

- Turn off the T.V, phone and all electronic devices at least 1 hour before you want to go to sleep, to avoid the blue light and unnecessary stimulation. There are blue-light blocking glasses that can minimise the impact that this light causes in our system throughout the day, which has been shown to affect our *melatonin* production (which is responsible for our natural circadian rhythm. This allows our body to differentiate when it is day or night)

- Exercise during the day to enhance endorphins within your system, but do not exercise within 90 minutes of bedtime, as it can work to arouse you too close to sleep. Gentle stretching or gentle yoga may relax the body, but try not to exert yourself too much prior to bedtime as it will have the opposite effect within your body

- Try to have a beautiful oil self-massage with warmed sesame oil (this Ayurvedic practice is called *Abhyanga* and is explained in detail later in the book) together with a warm bath with plant and flower essences, as well as magnesium as a muscle relaxant to calm the nervous system and pacify the aggravated *Vata dosha* (Ayurvedic constitution type comprised of the elements of air and space, which is explained in detail further in the book). Soothing the nervous system, particularly at night, may help to induce sleep as well as nourish your body after giving birth

- Stay away from caffeine in tea, coffee and chocolate, for some even as early as midday, though recent studies suggest 2pm is the ideal 'cut-off' time. Caffeine being a stimulant works to activate the sympathetic nervous system and disrupts the body's natural ability to fall asleep or remain asleep. Trial and error is the best way to recognise what time should be the latest that you consume it, without it affecting your sleep. My latest time is 4pm and beyond that, I will always reach for a herbal tea such as dandelion, peppermint tea or an Ayurvedic tea blend that my body needs for that moment

- Be mindful of eating very heavy, oily or fried food at dinner time as it may cause heartburn and indigestion. Try not to eat within 2 hours of bedtime as lying down can impede digestion, and alter the quality of sleep or ability to fall asleep. Sleeping with more raised or 'propped up' pillows may help with gravity for digestion, if you are finding that a heavy meal is affecting your capacity to sleep well. Listen to your body and the cause/effect dance that it plays with you and always trust your awareness of all the things you are noticing

- Try a guided meditation to help you redirect your thoughts and calm the mind. Beautiful healing soft music also can help, to soothe the nervous system and allow you to wind down before trying to sleep

- Essential oils can have queries with regard to their safety, due to their potency for use during pregnancy and in small children under two. If you are pregnant or breastfeeding or have your baby in the same room, then I would recommend you use natural plant essence infusion types, but utilising lavender, frankincense, chamomile, bergamot, neroli, rose, sandalwood, ylang ylang, myrrh and marjoram for examples, as they can help to promote or enhance relaxation and support sleep. Whilst this is not a dissection of clinical trials ascertaining the percentage of effectiveness, as the scientific mind would search for, these are plant essences that are anecdotally used for bringing calm to the system and may well be a simple and pleasant tool to add to your tool box

- Keep the bedroom dark and use an eye mask if there is light in the room. Weighted eye masks can help to soothe the nervous system also, as well as weighted blankets which have been utilised for anxiety in adults and animals alike. If sound is a disturbance, then use ear plugs especially if outside noise is unpredictable

- Journal or write down any constant or intrusive thoughts so that it is cleared from your mind before going to sleep, rather than festering on them throughout the night

- Have a herbal tea but not with too much liquid, so that you do not need to use the bathroom throughout the night. Think of chamomile, lemon balm, passionflower or lavender as warming and calming options. Even boiled milk with some turmeric, cacao, ghee and possibly cinnamon and/or cardamom with a touch of honey once it has cooled a little can also soothe the nervous system and calm the body to promote sleep; again not too much liquid to wake you for the bathroom

- Deep breathing or *Pranayama* (such as alternate nostril breathing) can help to relax the nervous system and calm the whole body down

- Do not do any other activity in bed other than sleep or intimacy, such that your body connects the bed to sleep and not eating or watching T.V. It becomes your sanctuary for sleep

WHAT CAN I DO WITH MY ANGER SYMPTOMS?

Anger is a common symptom with depression and also anxiety, as well as just being frustrated by the situation or how you are feeling. It is important not to place any judgement as to how you are feeling; it all is what it is and there is nothing to berate yourself about.

Again it is important to articulate how you are feeling to your doctors and allow them to give you guidance and strategies to move through your anger, as the source may be deeply imbedded or be a symptom that makes up the entire puzzle of your condition.

However, as a quick guide as to how to navigate your anger;

- meditation can be a very calming activity and allow your neural pathways to reconnect into being more calm in nature

- exercise is a great outlet; running, boxing or weight training as physical outlets. Yoga and more slow, flow, relaxing type of exercise can help to slow down your aggravated nervous system and promote more calm feelings

- journal your feelings and frustrations so that they are not festering, but are going out of your system, as it can be very therapeutic

- minimise alcohol, caffeine and illicit drugs as they can all create more anger, being very stimulating (or *rajasic* in Ayurvedic terminology) in nature

- reduce the amount of spices and chilli in your meals as these can add to the heat within your body; an Ayurvedic perspective of the kitchen pharmacy and the effects that spices have on our body and mind

- try to watch, listen and be immersed in more calming stimuli. Very aggressive or loud or highly animated stimuli can encourage feelings of anger and frustration within your system

- breathing; deep diaphragmatic breathing is very calming and can help soothe the agitated nervous system. *Sitali Pranayama* is a type of breathing, directed in through your curled tongue and out through your nostrils which can exert a cooling effect within your body, which is helpful if feeling anger and frustration

- always ensure that you are safe, your children and everyone around you is safe. If you feel uncontrollable or feel scared, then do ring Lifeline and contact your doctor and treatment team ASAP

QUESTION AND ANSWER SEGMENT

What is the first thing I should do if I feel something is not right with how I am feeling?
Tell your partner and if you feel able to contact your GP, then schedule a long appointment with them as soon as possible. If you do not feel comfortable or cognitively able to make the appointment, then let your partner or family member take the reins for you in taking this first step.

Following this, they can prepare a Mental Health Plan for you and refer you to everyone that you need, to form your treatment team.

What should I do if I feel my partner or a friend has post-natal depression?
If you feel like you are identifying symptoms in your partner or friend, then speak to them openly about how you feel they may have post-natal depression. Open communication with unconditional love, no judgement, kindness and compassion will allow you to navigate this delicate conversation with the respect that it deserves.

Do it without the distractions of chaos, noise and mess which can take away from the important conversation. Broach the topic with single pointed love and care, but not so it feels intrusive or accusatory per se. Make the time, set the mood and create a cosy space with a cup of tea with an ambience of openness and being able to create a welcoming conversation. No matter what their reaction is to your conversation, be kind and compassionate as denial or resistance may happen, but that should not deter you from keeping this beautiful woman safe and well. Planting the seed may be the first step into her healing so do not shy away from it.

When will I start to feel better?
This is a difficult one to answer, in that there is no magic crystal ball with a dedicated time frame for each one of us. Everyone has their

own unique foundation, biochemistry and factors involved so there is no black and white definitive time frame.

For me, I fell ill on day 5 for both children and recovered both times at 11 weeks post-partum. That is my experience but everyone can be different. However, having said that, taking your first step in reaching out means that you have taken the bravest step and that is the hardest part. Treatments can be worked through one at a time until you achieve the result that you require. How blessed we are to live in a time where so many treatment options and modalities are available to us.

It may feel exhausting and trying when there is no definite end goal; which I *fully* appreciate as being one of the things that I struggled with the most. Yet, I would encourage you to allow each treatment the opportunity and possibility to work amazingly well, as our mindset is so important and critical during our recovery. Focusing on what we don't like or have vs focusing on gratitude and having optimism have very different outcomes within the body, mind and spirit. Be open and allow yourself to receive the healing and have trust that you *will* start to feel better.

Should I get blood tests done at all?
It is not my place to demand anything from your doctor, however I do feel that baseline blood work is an important part in identifying other possible underlying conditions, underlying deficiencies or imbalances that may be corrected, in order to help you as a person in your entirety. It is well worth asking and finding out if anything is out of balance that can be corrected from the outset, and to treat you holistically.

Can I still breastfeed if taking medication?
All medications, herbs, spices, food, alcohol and drugs have the capacity to pass through the milk supply and into your baby. In terms of the specific medication chosen, it is important to tell your

doctor and pharmacist that you are breastfeeding as the medication chosen can be tailored to ensure that it is the safest option to treat the symptoms you have.

The simple answer is that you can still utilise medical treatments if you are breastfeeding, and breastfeeding alone should not be a reason not to seek treatment as there are a number of safe options to use.

Can I drink alcohol with medication or whilst I have post-natal depression?

Generally speaking, alcohol is a depressant and the medication that you are taking is trying to exert the opposite effect. Ideally, it would be best to avoid or minimise alcohol as much as possible so that it does not reduce the effects of your medication, nor keep you in the depressed state longer or deeper than necessary. It has been known to exacerbate depression and anxiety in individuals, especially if used as a crutch to mask the symptoms.

Alcohol can also enhance sedation, some side effects with medication and can potentiate or enhance the effects of medication, depending on which ones you are taking. There are some that you absolutely should not take with alcohol and others that may be safer. That is a conversation that should be had in detail with your doctor and pharmacist based on your individual situation.

I would also add the final point about alcohol - that it can be very taxing on your kidneys and liver, so drinking whilst on medication is putting your body under more pressure with the need for your organs to metabolise and clear both from your system, which may enhance the toxic load throughout your body.

What if I take other medication or over-the-counter medicines? Will it affect my medications for PND?

There is always the prospect of interactions with over-the-counter medication, including herbal supplements with any prescription medication. It is vital to discuss this with your doctor and pharmacist to make sure that timings can be managed and critical interactions be avoided.

This is where I am always mindful with herbal supplements as they can interact with various prescription medications. For example, St. John's Wort, when used for anxiety and depression symptoms, can reduce the effect of the contraceptive pill and interact with a few antidepressants, so it becomes ever more crucial to inform your doctor of everything that you are taking *prior* to commencing medication. If a patient did select it off the shelf after doing some Google research and was also on the contraceptive pill, then it could reduce the effects of the pill and she may conceive again whilst in the throes of PND. This outcome would be far more complicated than anticipated. It is always best to have transparency with your doctor, pharmacist and naturopath as to exactly what you are taking, so that no deleterious or even dangerous drug interactions occur.

Why do I have it when others in my family do not?

My older sister had three children and it did not affect her, so it is possible for this to happen. If you have it once it does not mean that it will happen again. For me it did unfold exactly in the same way each time, but that does not necessarily mean that this will be the same for you.

Whilst family have similar genetics and environmental factors to some extent, we are all unique in our blueprint and so whilst family history of anxiety and depression can be predisposing factors, it does not necessarily mean that everyone having babies will respond in the same way.

What do I do if I feel my treatment is not working?
It is critical to keep your prescribing team informed as to how you are feeling at every step of the way. Communicating how your sleep, appetite, mood and functioning are progressing, become crucial milestones as to how treatment is working.

If you and your family feel like your treatment is not working as well as you would like or hope it to, then please be honest and open with your communication about this. It can take 1 to 3 weeks for an effect to be seen and up to 8 weeks pharmacologically speaking, to see the maximum effects of a medication; though other variables within their psychotherapy may alter this time frame for your prescriber.

Open communication is the way to get to where you would like to be. It is also important to use your partner and family as a sounding board as to how your progress is, as they may have noticed a huge improvement even though you have not, or vice versa. Having a reliable and supportive network during this time can be so beneficial and helpful for your healthcare team, to know exactly how you are travelling.

Who can I connect with if I have post-natal depression?
Early childhood centres within your community health facility can arrange for you to join a group with post-natal depression mothers, similar to the standard mothers' groups they offer. I did not feel comfortable enough with my overwhelmed situation to attend such a group. I was in denial. I had it, and I could not cognitively function enough to physically get there and connect to people...however, each woman knows her own limitations at this time.

There are also so many PND specific groups on Facebook that you can join, if this feels more comfortable than face to face interactions. Chat with your child health nurse, GP or psychologist to connect you to people, if you feel that you are ready and want to do this. Remember you are not alone and there is so much support out there if you speak out about exactly what you feel would help you. Take a family member or your partner if you feel their presence would help you.

Does this mean that my children could potentially have this also?
There is a genetic possibility that your children may suffer from post-natal depression, given that a family history of anxiety and depression is a pre-disposing factor for PND. There is nothing to carry guilt, shame or fear about; simply an awareness that it may happen. Open communication to them when they are old enough is important and hopefully by that stage we have made leaps and bounds in our research and development into this.

Is it possible that I relapse or can have another episode other than after giving birth or in the 'post-natal' period?
If you continue your treatment as prescribed (whatever that may be); medication, to the CBT, IPT or MBCT, behavioural therapy or counselling, then I hope that you can manage your symptoms and condition throughout your motherhood journey.

The aim for medication is that it can restore any biochemical imbalance. The aim of psychotherapy is that it can navigate through trauma, get to root underlying causes, change behaviour and provide coping strategies to get through this chapter of your life.

Hopefully with being able to implement the strategies as well as restore biochemistry, relapse will not occur. Yet, it is always important to check in with how you are feeling at each point, be mindful of triggers, reduce stressors that may add any pressure and hardship in allowing you to remain in maintenance. If you feel that triggers or stressors are culminating and adding to making you feel worse, then lean into your triage team to give you further modifications and more strategies to allow you to cope with the revised changes. Sometimes it can be a work in progress; but similar to diabetes or a heart condition, it may require tweaking, alterations and management for as long as you need. There is not always a diagnosis, then treatment and a quick fix. For some yes, for others it can be a constant choreographed sequence until you get the performance right.

Sometimes I feel like with spirituality, mental health is similar in that you may never have 'arrived' at your perfection state. It requires healing, shedding, moving forward sometimes, and sometimes going ten steps back before moving forward again. It may not always be linear or sequential.

It is part of the process, but I feel as long as you are honest, you communicate, you are able to connect with how it is that you truly feel, find your most rock solid triage team and constantly remind yourself of your commitment statement, then you will have this!

Hold on and do not ever give up.

HEALTH TIP:

WHAT ARE AYURVEDIC NUTRITION PRINCIPLES
TO APPLY POST-BIRTH?

+ Eating warm, oily, moist and heavy foods (not fried or 'fast food') to nourish the body

+ Eating Prana (life-force) filled fresh produce (avoid leftovers, stale foods & processed food)

+ Eat regular meals especially when breastfeeding. Do not skip meals post-birth

+ Do not drink large volumes of water too close to eating (within 30 minutes) as it can impair digestion

+ Do not drink cold water or drinks; instead choose warm or hot drinks to aid digestion

+ Try to eat home-cooked food infused with loving intention and avoid raw or cold foods

+ Try to incorporate the SIX tastes of Ayurveda in each meal to create balance & healing;

Sweet, Bitter, Sour, Salty, Pungent, Astringent

HEALTH TIP: RECIPE FOR KHITCHARDI

This is a classic Ayurvedic recipe that is well known for its ability to balance the body, is easily digested and nutrients are assimilated in the body beautifully. It is a nourishing meal that can help bring the warm, oily, earthy elements that a mother needs after birthing her baby, which makes for a perfect post-birth meal!

INGREDIENTS:

2/3 cup red lentils or split mung beans

1/3 cup basmati rice

2 tablespoons Ghee or coconut oil (if vegan)

2 tsp ground turmeric

2 tsp salt

Half tsp fennel seed

Half tsp ginger powder or fresh ginger if preferred

1 tsp coriander powder

1 tsp cumin

1 small carrot

Half a sweet potato

DIRECTIONS:

1. Rinse the lentils and rice under water until clear then add into rice cooker with 4 cups of water (or depending on what your individual rice cooker needs)

2. Chop the vegetables (other root vegetables are perfect for this recipe!) and add to the rice cooker

3. Melt the ghee or coconut oil in a frying pan on a low heat

4. Add the spices and cook until they release their aromatic smell

5. Then add the spice mix together with the rice and vegetables in the rice cooker...then switch on!

Eat freshly cooked whilst hot and feel the nourishment that it gives to your body

CHAPTER 2

REFLECTIONS AND
TAKE HOME MESSAGES

During my time in reflecting upon my learnings from my post-natal depression, I was able to infer 24 different reflections or take home messages. Below is a quick reference guide and then I go in depth into each one throughout this chapter. My intention here is to allay any concerns or feelings you may be having about certain aspects, in the hope of it providing you with solace and peace about them.

Read all of them or skip to the ones that resonate with you the most.

1. How we birth does NOT matter
2. We need to be more kind to ourselves, whatever our breastfeeding journey looks like
3. Write a commitment statement to yourself
4. Drop the comparison
5. Research is required into definitive and underlying nutritional imbalances as pre-disposing causes for PND
6. Our identity after having children
7. Confusion of overwhelming information overload
8. Fear of getting into trouble or the implications of speaking out

9. Find your no-fuss friends and tribe
10. PND affects all those around you
11. Body image and self-love of our body after having children
12. Inner self-talk is important to monitor
13. Aspects of control
14. Releasing judgement
15. Releasing guilt and shame by speaking out and receiving help
16. Health is the most important thing and don't be deceived by what things appear on the outside
17. Ayurveda principles as a beautiful way to nourish and support a woman post birth
18. Importance of infant massage in our healing from PND
19. Need for a connective relationship in pregnancy vs clinical/ masculine approach
20. Dr Shefali's Portal of Pain theory
21. An opportunity to evolve and shift outdated paradigms upon healing to live my best life
22. Need for change and light
23. Listening to your intuition; your inner guidance system
24. Final Word

REFLECTION 1: HOW WE BIRTH DOES NOT MATTER

The way in which we bring our babies into this glorious world DOES NOT MATTER.

After my emergency C-section I was adamant that it was because of my significant amount of weight gain that caused a long labour and inability to have a 'natural' birth, which created a more intrusive or invasive means of birthing. I blamed all of this for causing my PND the first time.

However, with conscious mindfulness of optimal foetal positioning, undertaking Hypnobirthing, weekly antenatal yoga classes and remaining active throughout my second pregnancy until the day I did go into labour, I did have a successful, easy, effortless and joyous VBAC (Vaginal Birth After C-section). I felt extremely proud and felt very feminine as if my body had achieved what it was designed to do, in being able to experience a 'natural' delivery...but it *did not change* the outcome at all.

I will admit that the physical recovery and positioning for breastfeeding were easier with a non-intervention VBAC without a doubt. Hands down.

However, on day 5 after both births when I had the fall into PND, it didn't matter how I delivered my child at that point. My thoughts were not even about the method of delivery but more focused on where am I and how do I get out of this dark hole? Also when I could not eat a morsel of food or sleep a wink of sleep, the recovery made no difference at all as I lay in a foetal position in my bed devoid of any feeling or emotion.

In fact, if anything, because I had placed all of my focus on the labour and Kaiyaan's positioning that I didn't just allow myself to enjoy and 'be' in my pregnancy, especially towards the end as I was so fixated on the outcome. I was too concerned with how my tummy was reclined when driving, sitting and working. Towards the end I would watch TV whilst reclined forward so he would always be in the optimal position. What an exhausting waste of time and energy in hindsight!

I wanted a natural delivery so that I could drive after my delivery and not have that feeling of being trapped in the house. Yet, because of my state of being, I could not and did not drive for at least 8 weeks and even then, I would only drive 1km to my GP. It wasn't until I had recovered at 11 weeks that I felt confident and able to drive or felt like leaving my home for fun, so that reasoning was not actually a factor that was realistic in the end.

However, I also do know that if I had another C-section then I would have assumed that it was the method of delivery. Now, unequivocally I can say without a shadow of a doubt for me, that labouring in both ways did not control or affect the outcome of my post-natal depression. In fact, it certainly did not control the severity of my post-natal depression, as the VBAC had resulted in a *far worse* depression than my first, which completely disproved my theory.

I can also stand strong in saying that I felt no greater connection or bond once I had recovered from PND towards either of my boys. I felt their connection in utero and through the knowledge that they are a part of my being during my illness. However, I do not feel more close with Kaiyaan because he was birthed 'naturally' than compared to Ari. I love and feel connected to them now in the exact same way. My post-natal depression caused me to feel disconnected to both of them equally too, irrespective of how I birthed them into the world.

Because I had been so adamant about wanting to have a VBAC, my women's health physiotherapist who cared for me during my pregnancy, told me that doing too many pelvic floor tightenings could actually make a natural delivery more difficult. So, to be honest, I didn't do enough given that I so desperately wanted a natural birth.

I went to another women's health physiotherapist at the hospital after I had recovered from my PND to assess my pelvic floor and she reassured me that after 5 or 10 years (I can't quite recall!) that the baseline function of pelvic floors will realign irrespective of the way the baby is delivered.

In conclusion, having both a C-section and a natural delivery did not alter the outcome of having post-natal depression.

REFLECTION 2: WE NEED TO BE MORE KIND TO
OURSELVES, WHATEVER OUR BREASTFEEDING
JOURNEY LOOKS LIKE

We need to be more kind to ourselves whichever way our breastfeeding journey turns. As a health professional I knew of the message of 'breast is best' and I would always support my patients in best optimising their breastfeeding journey. I would support them through giving them up-to-date advice, discussing medications or herbs to stimulate milk production, as well as navigating their journey of taking medications/herbs/over the counter products whilst breastfeeding, as well as the safety of alcohol. I knew all of the gold standard information and guidance to give mothers, except it was to my own detriment on my own breastfeeding journey.

The pressure to be able to give my baby the best, fell heavily on my shoulders. We do our absolute best for our baby during pregnancy so I approached feeding with the same level of commitment and dedication. Yet, when I could not attach correctly despite having every midwife and lactation consultant available for every feed in the hospital and having access to them afterwards also, my milk supply was not stimulating. There was no adequate suckling due to technique as well as my heightening anxiety as each day passed. I would be bleeding from the nipples at every feed, even if I was only expressing. They both would scream at each feed and were losing weight which made me feel like I was absolutely failing. I felt this feeling of failure especially after Ari since I also had birth disappointment to contend with, so I felt very resentful towards my body not being able to perform all of these seemingly 'natural' acts that I was 'designed' to do.

Child health nurses and my midwife had suggested that breastfeeding hormones could be what was making me feel so unwell and so I felt hesitant to keep trying, thinking that I may stay in this state for even longer than necessary. Attaching my boys and expressing, also filled me with dread at each and every feed and made my anxiety so much worse. Dreading every 2 hours meant that 10-12 times a day I was not having a very successful time with my children and they were hungry!

The anxiety reduced my milk supply... and my milk supply worsened my anxiety. Laughable. It was not at the time though.

I now know that the onset of my breastfeeding hormones or the shift from pregnancy hormones to breastfeeding hormones *was* what had set my post-natal depression off, so I am glad that I had made the decision to stop feeding when I did; which could be why when week-11 rolled on, my hormones and biochemistry were able to restore as I had stopped quite early within our journey.

However, the desperate need and desire to breast feed my babies, given that it is so divinely feminine and deeply connective with our children and where they receive optimum and complete nutrition; made me feel like the *biggest* failure as a mother. The disappointment and pressure I had put on myself made me feel so awful!

Seeing other mothers feeding so easily and effortlessly was a trigger for me early on after having Ari, as it made me question my femininity and my ability to nurture my child. The pressure from social media, articles, the tag line of 'breast is best', all resulted in me feeling very inadequate and riddled with guilt, shame and resentment towards my body for not doing what nature had designed. Even being asked why I wasn't breastfeeding at mother's groups or by well-meaning people added salt to a very open wound; which is more a reflection of where I was at the time, rather than anything else. I also felt so embarrassed making formula in front of people as it was a reminder or a visual that I wasn't breastfeeding...and more so that I *couldn't* breastfeed.

I had to do a lot of healing work after quite a few months of this to heal those elements within me. I slowly learned not to feel embarrassed when I made formula for my baby and to feed him with the same love and intent as I would if I was breast feeding. I recorded my own guided meditation whilst feeding such that I would focus *all* of my loving energy and intention into bringing the divine light into his milk. This allowed for the process to be a more connected and heart-centred approach, rather than being riddled with emotional Ama/toxicity; an Ayurvedic concept of toxins/un-metabolised substances (or emotions) remaining in the system, and not assimilated or cleared. It changed my experience with feeding *completely* and I am so grateful that I recognised it and developed the tool to help me make peace with the whole situation.

With the birth of Kaiyaan I had joined the local ABA group whilst I was pregnant in the hope that I had armed myself with the contacts to assist me in breastfeeding after his delivery. However, because I had fallen into such a heap by day 5, I was unable to seek the help and assistance and stayed home trying to express and hiding from the world. Whilst I felt like I had my ducks lined up, the reality was I was unable to access the help because of the state that I was in.

There is also the pressure of not allowing the baby's weight to drop too much, the risk of jaundice from not drinking enough and the pressure of being labelled 'failure to thrive'. I also had lactation consultants and midwives saying the latch and attachment were correct and yet, Kaiyaan would literally take chunks off me and I felt like it was never healing and he was not getting enough milk!

After I had Kaiyaan I also had been prescribed Motilium which is Domperidone, which works by stimulating the release of prolactin, which in turn blocks dopamine, the neurotransmitter, as a way of stimulating milk supply as a strategy for my poor milk supply that I had with Ari. As a pharmacist I knew the pharmacology behind this and when my intuition in the hospital intervened and said 'no' to the nurse but stopped her before she left and changed my mind, I believe that was my inner guidance intercepting and yet, I didn't take heed. I delved into my treatment and gradually took higher and higher dosages as instructed and I believe that this surge of blocking dopamine catapulted my cascade into a further and deeper depression than had I not initiated therapy. As a trained professional I knew this theory and the method of action and yet, I wanted so badly to breast feed and have milk supply that it unfolded to my own detriment right before my eyes.

With Kaiyaan I was able to make peace with my feeding much sooner because I continued to add and listen to my guided meditation recordings as I fed him. It gave me an amazing connection and almost Reiki type essence in feeding him in his beautiful nursery. It felt like a very spiritual and connected time where I placed all of my intention onto him as I fed, and that has truly helped in healing this unfulfilled aspect of my journey.

I have created a recorded guided meditation designed from the one I used with my boys as a support tool for you to listen to whilst feeding, whether it be bottle or breast. It is a very soulful and connective process with your baby to be completely present with the feeding process. The idea is to fill the milk and process with the intention and feelings of love and nourishment, which is the *only* purpose for feeding. I hope this tool can help bring peace and solace if you are having trouble making peace with this aspect as I did. You can find this on my Wholeistic Healing Co. website and hope that you enjoy it as much as I did.

I now want to be the advocate for 'fed is best' and to remove the pressure that we place on mothers to be exclusively breastfeeding their babies. For those who can, I applaud you and I wish you all the success in your feeding journey because I know that what looks seemingly flawless on the outside, would have taken a lot of patience and perseverance. Fill your heart with so much gratitude towards your beautiful body in allowing this amazing process to occur!

For those like me where the hormonal constitution and logistically the latching/attachment/milk supply is just *not* working, especially with medication management, then let me be the voice of understanding, the voice of compassion and kindness. It is OK to not be able to continue your breastfeeding journey *if* that is what you choose or is best for you and your family. There is no shame in bottle feeding and I hope you find peace and solace in the knowing that by sending and feeding your baby with the intention of love, nourishment and nurturing, that your baby *will* thrive with the essence and energy that they are receiving, irrespective of the source of milk.

I am *so* thankful and filled with gratitude that we live in a world where milk supplementation *is* available and our babies can be fed and not starve, as they may in other parts of the world or in a different time of life. I say this because if I had continued to breastfeed as unsuccessfully as I was, I may have lost my babies through starving them, or the hormonal and biochemical cascade of breastfeeding could have worsened my PND or made my recovery even longer than 11 weeks.

I also want to acknowledge that for some women during the weaning process of breastfeeding, there can be an exacerbation of anxiety or depression symptoms where they may feel more centred and aligned when they are feeding. Suffice to say that each one of us has a different reaction to commencing, maintaining or weaning feeding; so be aware of *how* you are feeling and reach out whenever you feel less than optimal as to how best to navigate through that particular stage that you are in. Again, there is no-one-size-fits-all model of what breastfeeding hormones or weaning of these hormones can bring about to your individual system. Awareness and observation *is* the key here and being kind to ourselves throughout every stage of this journey is what is best for our body, mind and soul as well as our beautiful baby.

REFLECTION 3: WRITE A COMMITMENT STATEMENT TO YOURSELF

I believe when you have identified that you have post-natal depression and are ready to step forward into your recovery; the first thing I want you to do is to write a commitment statement to yourself.

Commit to taking whatever steps are required to heal, to do whatever it takes and write your WHY of wanting to heal. Knowing *your* why will help motivate, guide and keep you going each and every day into moving towards this goal even when you feel like giving up. This is your personal statement and it will keep you accountable each and every day.

Stick it on your mirror so you see it every day, place it on your bedside table or give it to your partner or family member so that you are constantly reminded of what an amazing life you have committed yourself to! Once you do this, I feel like you have made a contract into actively pursuing your best life and that will keep your motivation and resolve strong and high! That does not mean that you may not have hard days BUT it will make you rise up and face them head on, because you have made a commitment to yourself.

It can look any way that resonates with you and I implore you to go and grab your favourite notebook, pen and go and write that right now. Get your partner and family member to sit with you and support you through this step if you feel like you need it...and then see what magic happens when you commit to this first step x

REFLECTION 4: DROP THE COMPARISON

Another reflection I had was this idea of comparison and the toxic hold that it has over us. It has the ability to grab hold of us and bring us down to our knees with feelings of inadequacy, failings and not being good enough. These feelings can permeate through *every* cell of our being and have the opposite effect on our biology to healing, nurturing, kindness and gentleness to ourselves.

What is an interesting point to note, is that whilst we are in the depths of the darkest PND, how can we compare ourselves to anyone except our *own* versions of *our* best selves? How can we compare our day of survival and just literally getting through the day to a mother that has posted all about her GF, DF, RSF (gluten free, dairy free, refined sugar free) treats that she has made in her immaculate home with not a hair out of place?

Social media was a HUGE trigger for me and I actually did not use it for the full 11 weeks and switched myself *off* from the world. I could not handle seeing everyone's happy and perfect lives when I was hanging on by a thread. That was certainly my coping mechanism along with the fact that I was unable to form sentences to respond to messages and keep an open dialogue with friends. I could only carry a voice chat with family who had to hear my latest loop obsession. My need to cut social media was also stemming from not being able to actually engage in it and not only the triggers that it stirred up for me.

Body image comparison is something that comes up repeatedly after having children, that can be potentiated through using social media. The constant images of flawless and perfect figures when you may already feel vulnerable, may not help how you are feeling.

I would suggest that if you are using social media, unfollow people or stories that make you feel anything other than better or good about yourself after your time on it. Use that energy and focus in your own inner healing and recovery and turn your focus and attention away from anything that might make you feel stuck or worse than you already do. Remember you are seeing their highlight reel and you can do one too holding a perfect baby, but it would not show all of the wounds and how you feel inside. Remember that it is not always telling you the whole and honest truth, nor can you see how they are *truly* feeling from a picture.

I remember when we went for walks around our neighbourhood with our pram, walking our dog, Ari on his bike, me holding onto Chandi's arm because I had no energy to walk, coming out of our beautiful home with two luxury cars in the garage. People would smile at us most likely thinking that what they saw was picture perfect. The snapshot of looking like we had it all figured out and together.

Yet, on the inside, behind the material items or seemingly 'perfect things' was *so* much suffering, sadness, feelings of why is this happening to us? As I would hold Chandi's arm, I would be going over my incessant loop and parts of him would die a little more inside each time I went on my tangent. I would not wish those days or moments upon anybody. Yet, those smiling faces are etched in my memory as remembering that those people had no idea of our reality!

My point is; don't be fooled by images of perfection and grandeur when it may not reveal the full story beneath that. What you may perceive to be 'perfect' or better than your current situation, may not be the case at all. There are depths to stories far beyond what you can see on the surface, so do not get stuck into thinking everything is perfect in someone else's life.

If you feel triggered to feel worse by comparing yourself to others, then try to stop allowing those triggers to come into your life. If you want to feel connected to the world around you, then I would say for you to only follow people or groups that help your healing and make you *feel better*. Anything that is negative, grandiose or makes you feel further away from your healing *must* be turned off or put away.

Remember that you are a perfect being who came onto this planet to bring *your* own unique light and presence that NO ONE else can bring or replicate. Even though you are having a hard time right now, I promise that with the right nurturing, treatment and nourishment that you *will* get through this time and your light will shine even brighter than ever before. You will feel so connected to yourself, your place here on the Earth. Fill yourself with the self-love and belief that you so desperately deserve.

I loved Melissa Ambrosini's book *'Comparisonitis'* where she goes through so many aspects of comparing ourselves to others and how it is doing such a disservice to our own being and that we should not do it. If you have the opportunity to get a copy and are able to find some down time to read it then I would highly recommend it. I also love all of her podcasts so if reading isn't up your alley right now (I was not able to focus on a book during my illness), then listen to her podcasts. I have listened to some amazing guests on there and I always come out of it feeling like I have learned something new in my time with her.

REFLECTION 5: RESEARCH IS REQUIRED INTO DEFINITIVE AND UNDERLYING NUTRITIONAL IMBALANCES AS PRE-DISPOSING CAUSES FOR PND

My pharmacological background definitely harnesses my scientific thinking into trying to find out concrete predisposing factors for why *some* women have PND and others do not. I would love to see more clinical trials and research into *what* underlying biochemical or nutritional imbalances are present that can be screened for and potentially supplemented, with the hope of preventing or at least minimising the impact as much as possible for future women giving birth.

I feel that certain underlying and pre-existing nutritional deficiencies *may* pre-dispose our nervous systems to more imbalance, compared to those who do not have them. I underwent various biochemical testing after I had Kaiyaan, and some more quite recently with my Integrative GP. The tests shed some light on the fact that my genetic makeup and nutritive precursors were very plausible factors as to why I was predisposed to having PND.

Though some GP's may be sceptical and my hope is that more conversations, more research and light is shined on this subject, so that a more definitive and scientifically proven correlation be made. However, I share this because after copious amounts of testing were done, I was found to have the following imbalances which scientifically felt relevant to my situation;

- low magnesium
- low zinc
- low iodine
- low choline
- low B6
- low selenium
- gluten intolerance
- two mutations of the MTHFR gene (methylation ability of B group vitamins)
- Pyroluria (body produces excess pyrroles which affect the absorption of zinc and b-vitamins; though *extremely* contentious in the medical field)
- low tryptophan and low serotonin
- oestrogen dominance

- low morning cortisol
- low GABA
- high oxalates
- as well as two strains of bacteria within my gut from a stool
  sample

In essence there was a profound inadequacy in my body to absorb certain nutrients from my food, which I can truly see as potential factors for predisposing me to post-natal depression. These are not found in basic blood samples and not what my OB's were looking for in their regular screenings during my antenatal time. I would love to be able to have screening for all of these levels, as well as serotonin, noradrenaline, dopamine and possibly the levels of hormones for assessing the baseline that the mother has, prior to pregnancy or birth so that indicators could be recognised with reference to a predisposition to PND.

This may be revolutionary in the way we manage our women, if a definite correlation can be made of an underlying nutritional and biochemical imbalance that will hopefully minimise the onset or presentation of her symptoms.

For me, the switch in my brain flicked off at day 5 which took me into the vortex of darkness, and switched back on at week 11 post-birth. There was no doubt that the change from pregnancy hormones to breastfeeding hormones within my system was *what* triggered this profound effect within my system. There was a huge impact of this hormonal shift on the levels of my serotonin, noradrenaline and dopamine to have such a profound depression and anxiety.

Yet, I am so curious as to what made me predisposed to that switch flicking at that point. Was it my low levels of nutrition listed above, genetics or my own unique individual makeup that I just simply need to accept?

I came across Dr Oscar Serrellach's *'Post Natal Depletion Cure'* quite recently on Melissa Ambrosini's podcast and went on to read his book. He is a doctor and saw things in his wife after their children were born, as well as countless numbers of women in his doctor's clinic. His teachings were amazingly profound with his writing about the effects of certain nutritional imbalances and the implications they have on energy, vitality and healing post-birth. His findings reflected a lot of what I was seeing in my own biochemistry, and I would urge you to read his book if you get a chance. He has a wealth of knowledge and as a medical practitioner, his knowledge is comprehensive and profound in what he shares.

What I found also fascinating was that in my Ayurvedic studies I learned that if the *Vata* (the constitution within the body that is made up of air and space) imbalance is not restored after birth, then symptoms of *Vata* imbalance can occur even up to 5 to 7 years after having a baby. This can present with insomnia, irritability, depression and anxiety as all part of the nervous system, in amongst a plethora of other changes. Dr Serrallach also mentioned in his book that his patients would present even 5 years after having a baby with these symptoms and since it is more than 12 months post-birth they cannot be diagnosed as post-natal depression and yet, they were not performing at their full level of health and well-being. I would highly recommend this book when you feel ready and able to read without feeling overwhelmed!

This parallel was fascinating to me and allowed me to feel like the Eastern modality of Ayurveda, that concentrates on rejuvenation and nourishment of the mother to allow for inner balancing and healing after delivering a baby, can be used in *addition* to Western medicine to treat and heal any biochemical imbalances.

Going further into the understanding of this *Vata* imbalance, is that the *APANA VATA* (a sub-set of the *Vata* system) which is involved in the downward propelling when we give birth, can become *so* aggravated after we birth our child. We physically need to re-balance and pacify/nourish our *VATA* system with the opposing elements of *fire, water and earth* in order to restore and attain optimum well-being and health. By nourishing and rejuvenating our physical bodies with balancing these elements, we can best support the physical recovery after birthing our children.

When I learned this from my Ayurveda teacher in Perth, I got tingles all over my body as it was such ancient wisdom that answered my questions as to what happened to me from a different perspective. It enabled me to see how Ayurveda can be applied to help women not endure as much suffering as I did, and I feel *so* excited to be learning and applying this ancient Eastern knowledge in our modern Western world.

My hope is that the two together will allow for a more cohesive and synergistic healthcare for our women. To not just use one modality or the other but the two synergistically. Imagine if by utilising Ayurvedic healing practices whilst waiting for Western medicines and treatments to work, that it allowed for fewer symptoms and less suffering. I would have welcomed *any* respite at all in my darkest hour. Though I would not have had the initiative or ability to drive my own healing, I can only imagine what my other reality could have been if I was given or presented things to do and try, instead of sitting in my room alone like a hermit ravaged by my illness!

My hope is that we can pave the way forward for more clinical trials and testing, to ascertain the potential gaps in our biochemistry and nutritional health to help restore optimum levels and minimise such an occurrence in the first place.

REFLECTION 6: OUR IDENTITY AFTER HAVING CHILDREN

Another point of reflection for me is the concept surrounding our identity as women. This is multifaceted for all mothers, but for a mother with PND who already feels like she is harbouring thoughts of regret or lack of bonding and attachment to her baby, it escalates the confusion with her new-found identity as a mother during this time of illness.

Feeling vulnerable, self-conscious and under-confident without the benefits of the hormones of serotonin, dopamine and oxytocin to help one feel very nurturing and 'loved up', the pressure to know what the baby needs especially when that connection is not there, makes the concept of identifying *as* a mother very complex.

I struggled a lot with my confidence and trusting my nurturing ability, as I truly felt like my heart-centre had disappeared until at week 11 when I 'came back to life' as I call it. At that point I knew what my baby's cries meant. I felt connected to him and like I knew exactly what he wanted and I knew that I could provide that for him. I had the cognition to be able to handle it with poise and composure until I did work out what he needed. The more we did this delicate dance together, the more fun and choreographed our dances were and it was truly beautiful. Yet, before this, it was *completely* forced, no heart or connection was there and it almost felt like my body was there but it was an empty vessel with nothing inside me at all. So how *could* I identify as a mother? I certainly did not feel like one. I definitely did not act like one.

Having children even outside of post-natal depression definitely confers confusion in our identity as women, as we move from maiden to matrescence in so many areas. Going from a successful career woman who was independent and contributed to the household financially, allows one to feel like an equal. Yet, now looking after a new baby 24/7 it often feels like there is nothing to show for your time, even though you are working harder and clocking in longer hours than working outside of the home.

Not making an income does undermine our value of self-worth, which I feel is from cultural conditioning. It feels like we are not contributing in a quantitative measureable way. To compensate, you can often end up taking on more of the baby duties and household tasks because you don't go out to work. You may do all of the night shifts because you do not have a physical work place to show up to in the morning. This however, can add to building resentment as you are doing so much and are exhausted, without an income to show for it.

Often women can feel guilty asking for help or down-time when their partners are off from work, because they feel like they don't have a right to spend any money or have a break. It is definitely different having family support of aunts, uncles, grandparents, siblings around you as opposed to being a sole family without any help. I can empathise with this, as up until only 9 months ago we too raised 2 boys with no family support, and only moved back to Sydney with our family when they were 2 and 6 years old. We were 'on' as primary caregivers every day. Without question. We were everything to these little boys, which can feel relentless and the responsibility feels constant.

Equally, I am a firm believer of women having a strong financial foothold and self-empowerment, so that they never feel financially controlled by their partners and stay in a situation that they otherwise necessarily would not. For this to occur, then being independent and current in the workforce is also important to maintain.

I am so grateful and blessed that my pharmacist work has allowed me to be flexible with my working hours. It has truly allowed me to be the primary caregiver of our boys, whilst my husband and business partners worked tirelessly to build their corporate dream. Yet, working hard and saving money since finishing school, I had always been driven and equated my contribution to how much I could earn, especially using my brain and skillset.

Equally, those mothers who work full-time can also feel like they are missing out on aspects of their children that they so wish they could be involved in. This can harbour frustration and resentment of still having to work as if they have no kids, but go home to looking after kids too. It can feel like you are torn and exhausted by wearing so many different hats, and it can be a very overwhelming reality.

A lot of women even as they are doing a start-up business will often not send their child to day care if they cannot afford it or cannot justify the childcare fees. Yet, they work as many hours a day as someone who works away from the home. The pressure on women to be nurturing and connected mothers, as well as savvy career women is one where I feel the question of identity gets morphed. Whilst our children are young, to be a present and ever-giving nurturer and mother as well as an entrepreneur, I feel like something will have to give because there is only a limited amount of time in a day...though it may be very possible to do it all, if it fires your heart and soul. I admire and take my hat off if you are able to establish such a beautiful harmony between all the roles, which would be #goals to aspire to.

Triggers are far and wide, for all women alike, so living with a heart-centred mindset and being full of compassion, empathy, understanding and all round sisterhood will make our journeys through motherhood feel so amazingly nourishing. Let us celebrate all women and all of their choices.

It required a lot of inner work and making peace with being able to anchor into my role as the mother, nurturer, caregiver and encompassing the divine feminine energy that my boys needed. I also found further insight when a dear friend Sunita in Perth, who practices numerology and healings, recommended a book to me written by Jan Spiller, 'Cosmic Love'. It sets out your relationships with different people and looks at Karmic relationships and soul contracts. A bit woo woo, but I have always found this fascinating!

Yet, ironically for me, with my two boys and Chandi, my role *is* to be the anchor and rooted within the family unit, such that it gives them *all* security, safety and allows them to live their truth and their best life. For me, all of their roles are to bring joy and fun into my life and allow for me to step into my power. Knowing that I have this role for each of them gave me the inner peace in knowing that my stability gives them a big sense of family. Through contrast, when I was ill with PND I can see how derailed they each became when I was not well. Knowing this, has given me a huge sense of peace and a sense of connection to my divine feminine energy that I provide to nurture my boys, feminism aside.

The irony is that in my journey of motherhood, it derailed me and pushed me off course with my PND and yet, through my healing and daily life with my boys, it has created a new version of me that is aligned to my truth.

Through motherhood, I was able to find myself, and that has actually been far more rewarding than any issues I had grappling with income, identity and career. I stand grounded in the journey that I am living my divine purpose, and here with the energy and tenacity that I was sent to Earth to live by.

REFLECTION 7: CONFUSION OF OVERWHELMING INFORMATION OVERLOAD

My next reflection is the reality of the confusion of information available that can catapult us mothers, even well-researched ones into a heap.

In addition to all of my variables that I changed from Pregnancy A to Pregnancy B, after researching and reading I decided to encapsulate the placenta after birth as it 'supposedly' can help to reduce post-natal depression and increase energy. Though my OB was not convinced, he obliged and I had booked and arranged for it to be encapsulated after the baby's birth.

I genuinely felt like I was empowered and had taken *every* step to stop PND from happening the second time around. However, when I had trouble breastfeeding, some of the midwives would ask if I had delivered my placenta in full, as retained placenta can sometimes impair milk production. I had also been asked this question with Ari. Luckily my OB after Kaiyaan had shown me my placenta intact so I knew that it was not retained. Yet, with my hormones causing havoc and having so much trouble with my milk supply, I did not want to take my $400 capsules (cringe!) in case it confused my body any more into thinking I had placenta in my body and would affect my milk supply even further. They sat there on the shelf never opened or used because I did not want to risk making my situation worse.

The different information that child health nurses or midwives can give, certainly can confuse us mothers. I entered a Google rabbit hole many times about feeding, my capsules and definitely sleep! Not only is it addictive, overwhelming and *incredibly* time consuming, it takes so much energy to know what to do! I was so used to studying for an exam then passing, that this felt like I was being thrown new exam questions every moment that I had not prepared for. I felt very overwhelmed with this new gig. I thought that the birthing component was the hard part and now I get to rest...wrong!

My advice would be to seek support from your partner in helping with the research if there are certain things that you want to learn about or need help with. Parenting is a partnership and you should share the reading and learning together so that it takes the pressure off you, and can allow your body, mind and spirit to rest and rejuvenate as it needs after birthing your baby. Reading and researching tirelessly ends up over stimulating your already aggravated nervous system and can hinder your ability to fully heal. Also, if you are like me and found concentrating on information extremely difficult with the anxiety and depression symptoms, delegating will be a far more efficient and effective thing to do. You can then rest your body and mind knowing that someone is finding out for you, but you do not send yourself into a spin through the process.

Certainly, if it is safety and health directed, then seek medical advice. Otherwise find one or two reputable sites and do not read the others. Save yourself the time and energy of needing to know everything (hands up all the fellow Type A personalities!) and just be OK with knowing enough.

Trust me, with a two-year old that licks the floor, windows and kisses our doggy on the mouth, I stopped Googling a long time ago and just go with the flow! Perhaps life with two children has shown me that parenthood throws a million things at you, that we become more discerning as to what requires our attention and what is going to be OK as it is.

I do however, absolutely understand the hair pulling when it comes to sleep. I completely lost myself down the Google rabbit hole with Ari, my eldest, and I bought Tizzie Hall's *'Save our Sleep'* and my husband told me to throw it in the bin because it sent me even crazier than I already was (though Ari was sleeping better than me!) To be honest, both boys had terrible sleep-inducing habits with a bottle and/or dummy and were held to sleep. At the 4 to 5 month mark they would wake a good 7 to 8 times a night and I would often hold them to sleep in my bed just to keep them quiet as Chandi had to get up early for work.

At 6 months, I purchased the Sleep Sense solution by Dana Obleman online as recommended by a GP friend. Following her program for both boys, I took away the dummy and all sleep props and they slept like a dream in their own rooms! Ari took two and a half days to nail it and Kaiyaan nailed it by bedtime that first day! This literally changed my life and I can say 'goodnight' and both boys will sleep happily through the night...absolute game changer!

Before the 6-month mark with Kaiyaan, I told myself that it would change and it wouldn't be forever...so hang in there my beautiful Mammas! Sleep *will* eventually come and there is light at the end of the tunnel! Don't stress too much about it until they are 6 months and they can understand sleep associations a bit more. Equally, find the right system or methodology that resonates with you. What I tried may enhance overwhelm or anxiety for some women and families, so choose what is best for you and your family. Every one needs to do what is best for their family and what you feel comfortable with. I fully appreciate there are so many views and opinions on this, not to bring up a contentious topic but more bringing up the physiological need for sleep in your healing journey of PND.

With Ari I thought I would be stuck like that forever and never sleep a full night again, which felt very daunting! Yet, knowing my successful experience with Ari, by the time Kaiyaan had the same issues I knew what my game plan was and I knew that I would get through this sleep deprivation soon. Luckily for me, he was an even faster learner!

Definitely try to catch up on sleep when and how you can until you reach this point. Sleep is so vital for your healing and recovery, and I promise that sleep *will* return in your home.

REFLECTION 8: FEAR OF GETTING IN TROUBLE OR THE IMPLICATIONS OF SPEAKING OUT

My post-natal depression came on day 5 after birth and instantaneously I was filled with fear about what that meant. Like other families, we had child health nurses and lactation consultants visiting our home, having follow-up appointments with my obstetrician, paediatrician at 6-weeks as well as the immunisations starting. It was all so unbelievably overwhelming because I was not in my fully functioning state of being. It also felt like the enormous pressure of being 'watched' and judged at all of these opportunities; though a healthy outlook would see so many opportunities to reach out for help.

I felt like I was so out of my depth and my condition made me unable to talk properly, make decisions and my usual level of functioning was destroyed to an extremely basic level. A Type A personality, who thrives on being organised, punctual and dedicated to committing and executing whatever task I had set out to do, had been transformed into an absolute mess!

I dreaded the concept of child health nurses in my own home when I was so unwell and my main thoughts were those of absolute *fear* and feeling petrified that they would lock me away. It was such a visceral fear that deep in my being I knew these feelings and thoughts were not rational and yet, I felt too scared to speak up to strangers not knowing what steps they may take.

They started running through the *Edinburgh Postnatal Depression Scale* (EPDS) which is a self-reporting screening tool assessed by health professionals, as to how you are feeling and screens for the potentiality of PND. It alone is not diagnostic without a clinical assessment and it was presented to me on at least two occasions before my 6-week appointment with my OB. The fear of what *might* happen was so palpable, that I felt like I couldn't be honest.

I felt vulnerable.

I felt at risk.

I felt like a failure and like I couldn't be honest.

Whilst this may seem alarmist and extreme in thinking, when you are plagued with a biochemical barrage against your normal functioning of your synapses, this whole process feels far too intrusive and it can set you off on a trajectory filled with even more anxiety and crippled with fear.

What is my solution then, given that this screening tool can be very helpful to indicate that you should seek help? I would say that it is important to release the fear associated with it and to be completely honest with how you are feeling. Everyone is there to help you, so have trust in the process. If you feel frightened to speak up, then let your partner do it for you. Ideally, we need to have a system where we do not feel scared of the outcome, where we feel honoured and ideally see the same nurse or midwife to establish rapport, instead of being churned through different people each time and having to explain the situation at every point. Also if they knew who we were from the beginning then they could see a change themselves and be supportive as an individual, and not a case file that they are seeing that day.

Clear definitive support should be given by the birthing team as to where to go if you need help. Resources, contacts and a game plan should be given to all patients during pregnancy about what they can and should do if they find themselves suffering from PND.

I would also love to schedule interviews with some child health nurses, to find out exactly what the process is should someone disclose that they feel like they have PND and/or feel like self-harming. I would love to shed some light on the process and what exactly happens, so that if other women have fears about this as I did, that we can appease any fear around this.

The irony is, that my fear of losing my children was a sign of just how much I did love them. Despite how unwell I was, my basic primal motherly instinct was there, *irrespective* of *all* of the scientific explosions happening inside of me! This reflection gives me comfort now in appeasing my guilt and shame, so that I can stand tall in knowing that even in the midst of hell on earth, my focus was on keeping my family together.

My other idealistic hope is that of setting up a tribe or community of volunteers (or government-funded), where older mothers or grandmothers can check in and be of support to new mothers at home. They can help around the house, listen to how they're feeling and act as a non-judgemental stepping stone and referral to the next resources of help that they need, if these women do not have family or support from their friends.

Whilst this would be a delicate operation and the execution would be challenging, there is a need for such a service so that we do not lose women in the system. This can happen in the current model due to fear of causing too much trouble, fear of losing their children, fear of their partner not understanding what they're feeling, and need to hide it or for the fear of coming up on the radar.

These are real and actual feelings that need to be given a voice, so that we can provide reform. It will help our mothers speak out openly, without the fear associated with the implications that may be real or imaginary.

REFLECTION 9: FIND YOUR NO FUSS FRIENDS AND TRIBE

We ALL need honest, supportive and authentic friendships and tribe when we have children! No ifs. No buts.

I grew up in Sydney and moved a lot all around Australia after we got married, for our business expansion. After 11.5 years away we finally moved back to Sydney after the year that was Covid (explains it all right?!). Ari was born in Cairns and Kaiyaan was born in Perth, after first moving to the Gold Coast, so we had picked up and moved our lives three times since we'd married. All of my family and 'tribe' as I knew it, were in Sydney.

I was so scared to join the mothers group at 6 weeks for both boys as I was so unwell. How could I be bright and bubbly and make friends when I was a ball of anxiety, and my depression made me as dull as a door knob?! I didn't actually join until around 14 weeks after Ari and was able to connect with some lovely mothers there, that I still keep in touch with through Facebook.

In Perth, I was lucky in that I knew a lot of the kindy mums from Ari's day care, so I had a lot of people that I knew at his school. I remember one of the school mums noticed that I wasn't myself and said we should go for coffee but since I was in no state to organise anything, it never happened!

Yet, this one beautiful friend Julene, who is now one of my closest friends and reminded me of my sister, at one drop off was saying how she couldn't get out of bed for days, looked like rubbish and felt like it too after giving birth. It was only by her sharing her honest experience and being so raw, that I felt *so* comfortable in saying how I was feeling and how hard the whole thing was for me! Her bright, vibrant and exuberant energy to this day, has us in stitches with our conversations that are *so* honest and authentic about the reality of our days. She has been a real Earth angel with the gift of honesty and transparency that she has given me!

I am *so* lucky that I have a tribe in my family, so that I was able to be authentic in how I was feeling with my husband, parents, sister, brother and in-laws and *was* given the space to do so. I did not have to hide or sugar coat anything and could let all of my 'stuff' hangout! They were my rocks during my illness and I didn't have to filter or not be transparent in *exactly* how I was feeling. They were there *every* single moment of *every* single day, without any judgement, only with kindness and were my *absolute* life line for which I am so *utterly* grateful...my no fuss tribe!

We all need a tribe that we feel supported and honoured by. If you do have family support, then be honest with how you are feeling and let them in to your hearts and into your world.

If you do not have close family then it becomes so important to have no-nonsense friends, free from competition, drama or making you feel worse by making it seem like they have it all put together. We need honest, open and available friends on tap, and I would love to see communities of women being built with a true sisterhood feel behind them...where all mothers feel held and seen.

In a world with Covid now, I can only imagine the isolation, feelings of being alone and demanding everything you need from your partner; that is, if you have a partner *to* lean on. Ordinarily we could seek comfort from friendships and other people around us. I see you and I acknowledge this harsh reality of the current situation.

My advice would simply be to find your tribe, however big or small, it need only be reliable and supportive. Lean on them with *all* of your heart and *allow* them to be your Earth angel, *especially* if your family is away like mine was.

We are not heroic for doing it all and the saying 'it takes a village to raise a child' is the truest statement uttered by man. Find your village and become the Mayor!

REFLECTION 10: POST-NATAL DEPRESSION AFFECTS ALL THOSE AROUND YOU

Another thing I realised upon reflection, is that post-natal depression has a profound effect on so many people and sinks its teeth into all those close to you. I say this not to add to any guilt or pressure in your healing, but rather an acknowledgement of the rippling effects that it *can* have on your relationships and life as a whole.

I remember when Ari was young and I was ill, I would look into his cot whilst he was sleeping. I was just vacant, with this dark presence about me and not entirely sure what I was thinking or feeling. Interestingly I thought that by recovering at 11 weeks that he would have been relatively unscathed by remembering anything, especially since we never spoke about it in front of him.

Yet, when he was around three years old, we were going for a walk and he was holding my hand and said 'I remember when I was little you were sick and dark'. It *blew* me away because I didn't think he would have had the observation, knowledge or insight into seeing me that way. I did own it and explained to him what had happened, but it made me think that the absence of his mother bonding with him in those early days *did* leave an imprint. Again, not to make anyone feel worse than they are already, but rather realising that the impact *can* be great if we do not take action into our healing. If it continued for much longer or I remained in the state that I was in until he was much older, then he would certainly remember *so* much more than he did already, and who knows what imprint that would leave on him.

I feel like as a mother I was not there when they needed their mother the most. I now have been with them for everything, every day since recovering as a way for making up for lost time. I know how volatile and precious life can be, so I place value on being ever-present and connected to them. I am constantly working on being a great example by working on my flaws, being accountable for my feelings and reactions, and living a very live example of being mindfully present and responsible.

I have worked on creating a lot of audios with Listening to Smile through my platform, that have stemmed from the fact that Ari told me that he knew that I was 'sick and dark'. It is a way to offer healing and messages of love to your baby, when you are unable to give it to them yourself. I am creating the healings so that they feel connected, loved and wanted to fill in the void that the disconnection part of post-natal depression brings. I am creating them with the intention that they would be tools that I wished I had utilised when I was not well, but were not available.

Ruphus, our dog knew both times that I was unwell and was completely absent from life. Perhaps my body was in the home, but I had not returned with it for those 11 weeks. The full essence of me; my joy, happiness, ability to connect and feel had vanished completely into an abyss.

He went from sleeping in our bed on my pillow, following me everywhere and cuddling me whenever he had the chance, to not looking at me, not sleeping in our room or being in close proximity to me *at all*. It hurt, but to be honest I forgot *how* I even interacted with him with that heart-centre part of me missing. I knew in myself that the essence of me had disappeared and he knew that too. Animals can sense everything. When I did recover, Ruphus came back to me and came back to doing all that we did before. Like magic, he knew that I had returned and was so forgiving; which is another beautiful lesson to learn and see from him.

I also truly acknowledge the tremendous stress, strain and turmoil that it can create on your partner and in your relationship. I can only think of how many relationships that would *not* survive such a turbulent ordeal. The pressure cooker stressful situation of having post-natal depression with a newborn and possibly older child; adding the element of financial strain and the pressure of life in and of itself, is enough to push even a healthy relationship with strong core foundations to its knees. I will candidly admit that the strain during that time *did* test our patience, strength in relationship and brought out a lot of frustration and stress during that time.

I understand that for the partner, it can be *so* difficult to be the financial stability, be the primary caregiver of the children and unwell partner, coupled together with sleep deprivation and doing all of the domestic responsibilities at home. We are human and that strain can show in so many ways; frustration, anger, sadness and it can crush the partner themselves. Chandi had lost 8kg in those 11 weeks from the pressure of it all, yet we were lucky that he could pull himself out of our business for longer than what we had first intended.

We were *so* incredibly blessed to have our family support with us in our home, to help us with the practical household duties of cooking, laundry, entertaining the children and cleaning. They did *all* that they could to help, every single moment of every single day. Without this practical and physical help, I am genuinely unsure how we would have survived. We also had so much family in Sydney who were also able to check in on us and be our support, to help navigate us through this hard time when we needed guidance, the strength and courage to keep going one moment and day at a time. We are *eternally* grateful for that.

My heart breaks when I think of those families that do not have support; who may be new to a community or in the country and be *completely* overwhelmed with the intense reality that they are experiencing...whilst having absolutely no one to call upon in this crisis. Also for those women who have sick children, sick family members and for those who are in a domestic violence situation. How much pressure and feelings of helplessness can one person endure alone? It feels so cruel and absolutely rips my heart out.

My husband and I have had to do a lot of healing work together as a couple, to work through all of the residual trauma and pain left behind from that time. It requires honesty, being vulnerable and raw in identifying our feelings when they arise, and then taking the time to heal those emotions. Unresolved emotions emerge even when you least expect it, but we deal with them head-on so that they no longer have that hold and grip on our lives. The effects are far and wide during the illness, as well as rippling on for even longer than seems necessary. Healing is not always pretty and has resulted in lots of difficult conversations and moving through what we are thinking and feeling, as well as calling each other out on aspects we feel need to shift.

We communicate with honesty when we see something that we need to change and heal. It has fast-tracked our growing individually and as a couple; it is not always pretty, not always Instagram worthy but always evolving, which I am truly humbled by.

With this in mind, and acknowledging from first-hand experience the stress and strain that is caused by post-natal depression, I have created some healing tools and exercises (though not to replace professional counselling) for you to do as a couple. They are designed to help nourish, bring back connection, honesty and understanding into your relationship. We were so lucky that ours was only 11 weeks, yet for those that may endure this for longer, it is even more crucial to heal and be transparent about all of your thoughts and feelings. This is so that you do not harbour any resentment, anger or frustration at your partner, as these are all seeds for potentially breaking an otherwise strong partnership. You can find these at the end of the book and I hope you find them to be useful, even as a carer and family member.

For those of you that are lucky enough to have family or friends' support during this difficult time, it is a good opportunity for me to say that it is *completely* normal and natural for there to be moments of everyone not seeing things through the same lens. Everyone views life through a different filter. Their wisdom and knowledge are learnt from their own experiences, so having the same views on what action to take or reactions, is almost impossible!

The most important thing I would say, is that everyone's heart is in the right place. *Your* healing is their priority. If you are able to speak up about aspects that you are finding that add pressure or discomfort to your healing, then use your voice and share how you are feeling. If you are unable to share this information, or if you are a partner or family member reading this, then I would say no matter what your stance is, work together cohesively as if you are at work and make this as peaceful a process by becoming a united team to solve the situation at hand. There is *only* room for creating space for a peaceful recovery with *every* ounce of unconditional love and support for this beautiful mother in the centre. This will truly help her in her recovery.

REFLECTION 11: BODY IMAGE AND SELF-LOVE OF OUR BODY AFTER HAVING CHILDREN

Body image and this sense of 'self-love' and 'self-respect' that we have as mothers towards our bodies, can be hugely pressing along the road of motherhood. From this change that we go through from maiden to matrescence, our bodies change during pregnancy to house and nourish our babies, and then they change again after we give birth.

When I was pregnant with Ari, I gained far too much weight assuming that I would breastfeed it all away! I couldn't breastfeed and was mortified by the reality of what I had done! My next pregnancy, I was mindful and gained far less, most of which was baby and fluid so I 'bounced' back reasonably unscathed. However, I could not eat more than a mouthful of food during both of my post-natal periods, so I dramatically lost a lot of weight during this time. This was not intentional but a symptom of my anxiety and depression that I could not eat no matter how hard I tried. This however, placed me into starvation mode which undoubtedly affects one's metabolism.

The very act of growing two big boys left my stomach incredibly stretched, and ended up having an umbilical hernia after Kaiyaan, which I later had repaired. These changes in our bodies are profound, and someone with a very healthy body image prior to these changes may have an easier time making peace with this process. Yet, if someone who was already riddled with some harsh views of her body, then she may have a harder time accepting and adjusting to all of these very extreme changes that happen with this creation process.

This leads me to question as to what effect does this constant 'yo-yo' change of weight, have on our system and the feelings involved with true healing at an inner core space, as to having an unconditional love affair with our body? We, as women, can be so harsh on ourselves and are our own biggest critics. Denying ourselves of this deep inner-self appreciation for our body, stems from a place within us of not being worthy or good enough exactly as we are.

We compare ourselves to others and feel bad about ourselves, or wish that we could change aspects of our body in a very critical or resentful way. I felt resentful for my body not being able to birth my baby the first time, and also for not being able to breastfeed given that it is such a 'natural' process. Those feelings took a long time to shake and be replaced with forgiveness and appreciation, for all that it *did* create and achieve.

In my studying of Ayurveda, I came across a principle or governing philosophy that forms one of the bases or foundation of all disease and illness... and I dare say *all* of our feelings of inadequacy or low self-esteem. It is in Sanskrit, *'Pragya Aparadha'*, which means the mistake of our intellect. It is the mistake of our intellect in remembering that we are divine, and is the loss of this knowingness within our mind, body and soul. It is this premiss, that we forget that our source is the divine itself, and so we make lifestyle choices with our mind that in turn cause even more loss of knowingness, that causes us to make more decisions and choices...that cause us to forget this fact even more! It is the loss of knowingness within our intellect that causes us to make choices that affect the qualities or *gunas* of the mind.

The aim in Ayurveda is to encourage our mind to increase in *Sattwic* quality (pure, balanced, harmonious, peaceful and virtuous quality of the mind) through practices and lifestyle habits. By increasing this quality, in turn we make more conscious life choices which in turn serves our entire being to remember this divinity within, as well as live in our most optimum state of health and vitality. I absolutely *love* this.

It resonated so much with me because it felt like *if* we remembered *our* source of divine wisdom and presence; that *we* are in fact a drop in the same ocean, then *how* can we ever think or feel that our body or ourselves are anything other than perfect? How *can* we think any thoughts to self-deprecate ourselves, and not just be in absolute awe of our amazing bodies? If we could appreciate being so divinely feminine, and connected to our creative bodies, that are a vessel and a gatekeeper for beautiful souls entering into this Earth, how liberating would that feeling be?!

Every thought that we make has a feeling associated with it that permeates to *every* cell of our being. Thoughts of anger, frustration, resentment, hate are all vibrating at a lower and constrictive frequency, that at a cellular level no doubt can give rise to dis-ease. Louise Hay has a whole book titled *'You can Heal your Life'* that I read even as a small child, as I have always been interested in the mind, body and spirit connection. It contains parts of the body that carry dis-ease due to feelings of a certain nature. She goes in depth as to

151

what emotions can create what illnesses within our system. Through awareness, letting go and affirmations from a feeling place, not just word space, it is possible to release deeply embedded belief systems and change the trajectory of your healing. If you have not read it, then I would highly recommend it!

We need to send love to our younger self and get her to love her body in its perfection and to love it through its *whole* journey; warts and all. We need to teach our sons and daughters that sending hate or ill feelings towards our vessels, is *not* going to make for a beautiful ride...it will be bumpy and turbulent instead of being smooth and joyous! We are set to fail when we start off by not loving our bodies, then end up feeling horrible when they do change even more after having children!

Thoughts of love, compassion, forgiveness, understanding and empathy have a more open and expansive feeling within our bodies. Imagine the effect at a cellular level as to what *this* will bring about in our bodies!

Whilst I acknowledge that the way in which we view, speak and feel about our body is so important, and that we need to embrace an all-encompassing love and appreciation for our bodies, that it is so much easier said than done. Thinking it on a logical 'word' plane, is so different from believing and practising it from an inner knowing and belief system. I am ready to break the shackles of my limiting beliefs and to honour, love and nurture my body as she deserves, and to FEEL it in an organic way and not a logical 'I need to' way.

I have started working on a 6-week program with Diana Fischer from *Body Positive Mama*, who I met by chance at a women's circle in Perth. She does such amazing work and her whole platform is centred around body positivity for women and we have been unravelling this portion of myself. I am *so* ready to heal and transform and I would highly recommend her as she is such a beautiful, kind, soft and nurturing soul, who has already helped me in making amazing shifts in this realm of my life. I am noticing shifts in how I feel, and am being more kind to my body than I ever have before.

Tomorrow is not promised, so live unapologetically loving every cell of your being! Easier said than done, but oh SO important!

REFLECTION 12: INNER SELF-TALK IS SO IMPORTANT TO MONITOR

Another thing that I learned to observe and modify during my recovery process, was the way in which I spoke to myself. The inner self-talk that permeated every conversation in my head, through *all* aspects of my life. How can anyone tell you that the way you perceive life or speak to yourself isn't serving you, if there is no sounding board to give you feedback. You don't know what you don't know, until you do! Then, you are able to check in on yourself and steer the ship in the direction and way that you want it to travel.

There is no doubt that my inner self-talk and conversation WAS critical, negative, riddled with self-doubt, thinking the grass was greener on the other side, very much a victim mindset of placing responsibility or blame onto others or situations, rather than claiming my power or even seeing it.

Our mindset, which I discuss in more detail in chapter 3, can either be 'fixed' and therefore limiting, or it can be an expansive and an 'open' mindset, which is focussed on growth and self-evolution. Compare being stubborn vs being flexible, controlling vs surrender, pessimistic vs solution focussed and learning focussed.

These are imprints that are set in our formative years, up until the age of 7, where we set the tone of *how* our inner-talk is governed. My childhood was one of being resilient, maturing early and so can see where my mindset set in. No judgement. Simply reflecting and having the awareness of where the seeds were sown, to be able to stand into my power and rise through and above them.

It makes me so mindful, that now I am the same age as my parents were when I was growing up, that of course they had their 'stuff' to work and navigate through, just as we do as parents. It makes me very much connected and aware of how I navigate my conversations through the day when I feel stressed, tired or overworked. How I voice those feelings shouldn't become the inner voice of my children growing up. They watch and imitate all that we do, so it becomes even more important to steer our ship into waters that we want our children to be proud of, and in ways that serve all of us to live our best lives.

I am very much aware of my anger, frustrations and feelings of stress that arise from the reality of balancing work, children and life; so have created audios that I put on to help centre myself and my children, so that I can re-set the frequency at which I am operating.

In the throes of post-natal depression, whilst I could observe critical and self-sabotaging inner self-talk, it was once I had come 'back to life' that I was *truly* able to transform and stand into the self-talk that I wanted to have with myself. Whilst analysing and working through it in the depths of your illness may create more overwhelm, you can revisit this aspect when you feel ready.

It is a continual work in progress and one that requires an open heart of compassion, rather than judgement. It also requires standing back and observing our thoughts, and is quite an empowering experience. We can realise that our thoughts are separate to us and not who we *truly* are. Thoughts can be changed and we are the real self beyond the thoughts and emotions.

Watch. Observe. Align them into where you want them to be, and how you would want your children to talk to themselves. I would imagine it would be in a way that is kind, compassionate, unconditionally loving and understanding. It is *never* too late for anything and we can take the reins in every aspect of our lives, in whichever direction we want. We have that much power.

REFLECTION 13: ASPECT OF CONTROL

I will be the first to admit that I am a Type A personality who likes structure, order, being organised, in control, task-centred, productive, ever evolving and growing! I sound like fun to live with right?! These skills, values or traits have served me in many aspects of my life. Yet, parenting and motherhood has certainly made me check in on this paradigm of *control*.

I felt very thrown in the deep end after having Ari and felt like I did not know what I was doing. I felt very much like a duck out of water who had not been trained in a new CEO position of a company, and felt *so* unbelievably out of my depth. It felt like I needed to know what my baby needed and wanted and I did not have any idea what I was doing! Again, a totally natural and normal feeling after your first child, as I did not feel *so* overwhelmed with my second child.

Yet, with my second I was being very controlling with my VBAC outcome. Whilst I would say I was surrendering into the process and what is meant to be will unfold, I made sure that I did everything humanly possible to ensure that I knew in my heart of hearts that I had done all that I needed to do, and could not look back and say 'I wish I had done x, y or z'. That though was pure 'control' disguised in the hat of action and 'empowerment'. I crossed every T and dotted every I, yet what if I didn't end up having a VBAC? Would I have been OK with it not going according to plan?

Parenthood has taught me that we can have the best laid plans and it sometimes just does not work! Running late and someone needs to do a poo. Cleaning the house and the boys destroy it whilst 'playing' or eating and leaving crumbs where ever they feel like it. Sound familiar? Yet, such a beautiful lesson in relinquishing that element of control and just purely going with the flow. Not sweating the small stuff. Business too has taught us to relinquish our control. It has been a huge life lesson into trusting our intuition, making a decision and being happy with the outcome knowing that we made it with the information and feeling that we had at the time. The outcome is out of our hands.

The first lesson of motherhood in the arrival of Ari, right there in those 4 minutes past midnight into him birthing on Friday the 13th, was that I could not and *should not* ever think that I can control this boy and his destiny at all. He is his own soul and being and has the right to completely live his path and not what *I choose* or *tell him* to be or do. A very humbling learning amongst many more I learned and will continue to learn throughout my motherhood role.

I know that we cannot control who our children become, what they do and what actions they take in various situations. This leans towards Dr Shefali's *'The Conscious Parent'*, which I implore you *all* to read and follow! Her teachings are phenomenal! It is all surrounded by letting go of control of our children, being present and teaching them not from a place of our inner wounds or holes, but to allow them to be who they truly are. Definitely worth reading and devouring all of her amazing content!

My advice at this juncture would be to find the true core values that *you* believe in. Focus your attention on living your fullest and best life in alignment with these values, without expecting others to follow in the same way. Live without control of any outcome and just go with the flow of life. How easy life would be going with the stream instead of against it? How effortless would life be if we breathed and truly surrendered, knowing that the outcome will always be for the highest good, so why try to change it?

Try as I might with everything, I attempted to change not getting PND the second time and yet, it eventuated anyhow. Not just that, but it resulted in the emergence of my voice, my authentic self and taking off a mask that no longer served me. Was it the hardest chapter of my life? Absolutely. Would I change it given the transformation that it did allow? Never!

REFLECTION 14: RELEASING JUDGEMENT

I have spoken a lot about the word judgement and it rings as an important aspect in many respects. The fear of judgement I feel holds so many women back from speaking out about their need for help. Judgement they may believe will arise from their family, partner, their doctor, other mothers but *especially* the judgement that they place on themselves. We judge ourselves *too* harshly and are our own harshest critics when we do not feel the way we 'should' or believe others do. Judging what we are feeling as being 'bad' or 'not acceptable' may keep us stuck in how we are feeling even longer than necessary, by not reaching out for the help that we need.

Be discerning with who you are sharing your deepest feelings with and ensure that they are creating space for you to be vulnerable. I feel like social media has given a faceless platform for so many people to comment and judge, without an understanding of the situation with unconditional love. This can be hurtful to the recipient, so it becomes more crucial as to what input you are receiving and who it is that you share your deepest feelings and situation with. This will ensure that you are in safe hands that will hold you with only compassion, openness and kindness.

Judgement comes from a space of an 'inferiority complex' or feeling less than, or having a 'superiority complex' or feeling better than the other person or situation. Without this judgement there would be space *only* for kindness in one's heart, empathy and compassion. Be mindful of your inner self-talk. Be kind to yourself. Always.

REFLECTION 15: RELEASING GUILT AND SHAME BY SPEAKING OUT AND RECEIVING HELP

Being articulate, authentic and not shying away from all of my feelings has been pivotal in my healing. By being able to articulate *every* thought that was ruminating through my head, there was no hiding or room to guess what state I was in to my family around me, who were able to steer and guide me into taking action every moment of every day.

I realise that we are human and it is OK to feel, *however* it is that you feel, but there is a line between what is 'OK' and what is not. It is 'OK' to have hard days of parenthood with the noise, chaos, mess and feeling tired or touched out. Yet, through experiencing the contrast of the darkness of PND I know what it feels like to not feel like yourself and for those days with suicidal ideations, those moments are not OK to be experiencing.

However, by feeling trapped in the dark thoughts and then hiding behind a veil of shame, guilt and fear, this is what can keep us back from walking into our recovery. There is NOTHING to hide. Remove the mask of pretending that you are OK if in fact you are not feeling this way at all. Remove any shame or embarrassment that you may feel and I hope that we can provide an open and safe environment for *you* to reach out for help.

I would love for all employers to know that if someone has had a baby that they may not be OK. Partners shouldn't have to feel the stress of keeping finances together, keeping up the level of work output at the same level as when they did not have children, and then looking after the children and a sick wife, as that pressure can crack them too.

Give them slack and ask if they need time off. Do they need help? If you run your own business, speak up to your partner and don't be a hero. Don't hide behind a mask whilst your whole world is crashing around you. Remove the guilt of asking for help and accept it with arms wide open, in the knowing that they are creating space for you to feel held and heard.

You do not need to venture through this alone. Fear, guilt and shame are what hold us back from our recovery. Yet, through being open and honest and accepting their hand in carrying us to wherever it is that we need to travel, in order for us to be able to heal is *complete magic*. Let this person or people be your Earth angels and carry you towards your healing. The sooner you get there the sooner you can put all of this aside and live the most amazing life with your family and children.

You deserve it.

REFLECTION 16: HEALTH IS THE MOST IMPORTANT THING AND DON'T BE DECEIVED BY WHAT THINGS APPEAR ON THE OUTSIDE

Another reflection is the concept of not believing everything that you see. What may appear to be perfect from the outside and may make you feel poorly about your own situation, is only a snapshot and not depicting the entire picture. Not because anyone is purposely trying to deceive you but because beneath a smile or a picture, no one truly knows the depths of pain or torture that may be happening moment by moment.

At the time that we had Kaiyaan, our corporate dental business was thriving in a way such that Chandi could extend his leave from two weeks up to six weeks when I was so unwell, without a blip on the radar. It served us in providing flexibility, freedom and a whole extra body to help carry us through this difficult time, for which we will be forever grateful.

At that time, we had established ourselves quite well and which to most, including us at the time, would be #goals to aspire to. Yet, during the time of my illness, none of that meant a *thing*. Literally. We would have done anything to bring me back to life and restore my mental health and well-being, if someone had a magic ability to do that for us.

Without health, any worldly possessions or 'success' mean nothing and once health is restored, it becomes *impossible* to place value or importance on material things and what 'happiness' you think it will bring you. I choose health every time. I choose mental health every time. I choose presence every time. I choose love. I choose living with an open heart and being of service. Every time.

Don't get me wrong, my heart is filled with absolute gratitude that financial freedom *did* allow for me to receive timely and high quality care to bring me into my wellness. It allowed me to be able to take the factor of finances away and expedited my access to services when paying and booking my next appointment with the specialist. I am proud of our hard work and sacrifice moving all around Australia, to even rural parts where most people would not go, in order to reach a place where finances in my healing was not a variable to consider. Yet, the reality is that *no* amount of wealth can bring you happiness and if you feel that others are happier because they have nice things on the outside, it is not the right conclusion to draw.

So it makes my heart break that for those women and families where each appointment would send them further into more financial stress. This factor in itself can fill you with guilt in needing such care, and you may not be able to see treatment to its fruition, which is very distressing. Not being able to pay gap payments after Medicare for psychologists can be a *huge* factor, and my heart goes out for this reality. My genuine hope is that quality healthcare becomes available for *all* mothers.

I LOVE the work that the Gidget Foundation do where they provide access to bulk-billed psychologists and care under their services, including Telehealth (remote services) and what amazing work this is! I want there to be more access and reach for these services, more funding to allow for Gidget Houses to be set up all across Australia, because this work is crucial in allowing women to seek and access government funded mental health treatment, at a time when their bodies are healing and they need this care to be as easily accessible as possible.

I am a Gidget Angel and my story is shared on their website as a commitment to spreading my message as far and wide as I can. The hope is to enhance access to services in as many locations as possible, as well as advocating for speaking up and getting the help that is needed to recover. I do not want families to suffer any longer than they need to, or to think that it will get better on its own or that treatment won't change how one feels, as I had thought.

My heart explodes when I think that it is not just Australia that needs this work and access, but the *whole* world! I think of the mothers in poor living conditions here, Africa, America, India and England and if they cannot access affordable treatment and support, then how many lives are we losing to suicide? I shudder at the thought of what the true figures are and not just reported statistics, because *how* many people are getting lost in the system to this truly all-encompassing illness? I am not entirely sure of what each country has set up in terms of services, but I would love to see that services are available so that reaching out for help is met with *so* many options. I want every woman to have the opportunity to move forward towards their recovery...their children and family need them.

I digress! My point was that I do 100 percent acknowledge the importance, value and place that finances play in a woman's recovery at this current place of life; and hope that we can create change such that it is *not* a relevant factor in the standard of care available. However, once mental health was restored it became impossible to place importance on material wealth as being a source of happiness, when despite having it we still endured so much suffering.

We would choose health and mental health every single time. Without the clarity, focus, fully-functioning mind, there is no way that you can feel any emotion let alone place any value onto anything material again. Do not feel trapped in thinking that happiness lies in something or somewhere 'over there'. It lies here in the now with your present day awareness and stepping into your recovery. Then you can fully savour your time here with your children, imbibing strong mental and physical health.

I also acknowledge that when Covid-19 first entered our world and we had our first lockdown last year, our business stared down an *enormous* amount of stress. We had supply invoices without any dentist production, given the restrictions that were instated in dentistry. There was financial stress in unknown waters and no knowledge of when it would end or how we would survive.

Yet, with our mental health intact, we could look the issue in the eye and go into solution mode as our Type A personalities know and thrive upon. With a clear and healthy mind, one can utilise the resilience and inner strength from within, and have the resolve to overcome challenges. Without mental clarity and health, it took me an hour to choose an outfit or 45 minutes to make a bottle. The contrast is clearly visible.

REFLECTION 17: AYURVEDA PRINCIPLES AS A BEAUTIFUL
WAY TO NOURISH AND SUPPORT A WOMAN POST-BIRTH

I know that I have mentioned Ayurveda several times already
without fully explaining it in detail. During my studies of Ayurveda,
I found that the knowledge and understanding of our *doshas* (energy
patterns within our body) and what happens to our balance within
our bodies after we give birth, were so profound in giving me an
understanding that filled in a lot of blanks of my Western medicine
knowledge.

For those who may not know much about Ayurveda, it is an ancient
wisdom of practices of medicine and life, dating 5,000 years back
to 3300-1300 BCE. Its literal translation from Sanskrit, means the
'science of life' and is based on the premiss that everything that
exists in life is made up of the five elements namely; air, space, water,
fire and earth. It is the combination of each of these elements that
gives rise to certain constitution types, each having their intrinsic
qualities. There are three main *doshas; Vata, Pitta and Kapha* that
make up your *Prakruti,* or your natural constitution that you were
born with.

The *Vata dosha* is made up of the air and space element and
comprises mainly the lower part of the body, though is responsible
for movement across the whole body. It has the qualities of being
cold, dry, light, mobile, rough, subtle/clear, hard and flowing. It is
considered the King or Queen of all of the *doshas.*

The *Pitta dosha* is made up of the fire and water elements and is
responsible for the process of transformation and governs digestion
as its primary role and centred around the torso region. It has the
qualities of being hot, liquid, light, flowing, clear and sharp.

The *Kapha dosha* is made up of the elements of earth and water and
comprises the area of the skull, chest and upper respiratory system.

It is responsible for protection and liquefaction and has the qualities of being cold, wet, solid, heavy, oily, dull, soft, static, dense, cloudy and smooth.

Knowing one's body constitution or *Prakruti* can be very helpful in making choices of diet, lifestyle and practices that best support the make-up of your body and allow for it to live in optimum capacity. Our body constitution can be made up of one or all three of the *doshas;* with being bi-doshic as the most common occurrence. I have a *Vata Pitta* makeup within my body.

The theory of like increases like, forms the foundation of Ayurveda such that we choose food, spices, herbs and practices that restore balance by exerting the opposite effect. For example, an aggravated *Vata dosha* which may present as insomnia or anxiety caused by too much air and space aspects in life (from a busy stressful lifestyle), can be balanced by bringing qualities of its opposite; namely heat and oiliness to bring about the earth, fire and water elements such as through a warm oil massage, *Abhyanga*.

The preventative mindset of wellness is inherent in this modality and believes that health can be maintained and restored through the application of diet and lifestyle practices. It encourages a holistic approach of utilising the mind, body and spirit components of life, to which I personally have found pivotal in my belief system. As a young girl and even to this day, I would draw in my diary a triangle with mind, body and spirit written on each length and then write how I would nourish each of these aspects throughout the week ahead. Ironically, Ayurveda teaches how to nourish each of these branches as a way to best support you in your health and vitality.

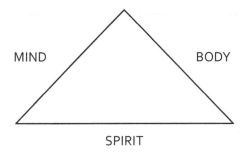

Ayurveda believes that what a woman eats, consumes through her senses and energy system, her lifestyle practices and mindset, *all* have an imprint on the growing baby in her womb. Mothers are then treated as divine goddess beings, the gatekeepers of creation and life, and are encouraged to nourish their bodies, as well as not be subject to stress and strain. I love the spiritual focus towards pregnancy and find it very beautiful, rather than a clinical process of life.

Ayurveda also explains the process of childbirth as the downward motion that can give rise to an imbalance (or *Vikruti*) specific to our *Prana Vata* and *Apana Vata* system; which are *sub-doshas* or sub-systems within the *Vata dosha*. As a result of this huge imbalance that results from the downward expulsion of our baby during childbirth, it can disrupt our whole *Vata* system and give rise to a multitude of symptoms because of the excess of the air and space elements; given the void within our womb after birthing our baby. These symptoms of imbalance can present as; anxiety, depression, insomnia, essentially an aggravated nervous system, erratic movements and inability to switch the mind off as some examples.

I find this parallel so fascinating as to what such an imbalance can cause physically in our body. The symptoms absolutely matched what I had and the 11 weeks was technically the fourth trimester, which in Ayurveda is the most sacred time to focus on rejuvenating, nourishing and restoring balance within the mother's system.

Coincidence? I think not. Ayurveda strongly encourages 40 days of rest, incorporating certain practices, herbs and nutrition to support the re-establishment of balance within the *Vata dosha*.

As an Australian born Indian woman, I gawked at what my parents would tell me as being old wives' tales. I could not understand why I should follow them arbitrarily without knowing how or why to do them or what benefit that they would bring me. Only through studying have I gained a full appreciation of their value and merit within the healing process. I believe that my role is to re-ignite their use in the modern world with full explanation as to how they work, so that we do not lose or dilute this ancient wisdom as the years go by.

As mentioned earlier in the book, Ayurveda also explains that if our *Vata dosha* is not balanced after we give birth, then we can present with symptoms of *Vata* aggravation in the form of anxiety, insomnia and depression even 5 to 7 years after having a baby. This similarity also parallels with Dr Oscar Serrallach's writings in the *'Post Natal Depletion Cure'*, where he states that he often saw women come into his practice 5 years later with these type of symptoms.

Therefore, I believe that utilising this Eastern modality in treating the woman through nutrition, practices, herbs and nourishing their minds and souls as well, in *addition* to Western medicine, we can holistically hold the woman and walk her through to recovery in such a beautiful and respectful way.

I believe that I am well placed to bring these two synergistically to encourage healing from both modalities. Teaching and providing the lifestyle practices to support *Vata* imbalance, guiding Ayurvedic nutrition and diet as well as guiding through the use of Ayurvedic herbs and spices in the kitchen as well as through teas and drinks. I am passionate about going back to basics of pharmacy and offer a more apothecary-type experience. In a busy and modern world, I believe that internal healing and wellness is the key to long-lasting health and vitality.

I am so grateful that I stumbled across pursuing my further studies, as it has resonated with my soul beyond belief. I knew that I was in search of my dharma, yet looking for it with logic and the mind was no way to find it. Through experiencing life and going through the journey step by step, putting one foot in front of the other, I have been able to connect with it through my heart space and through contrast of how it feels, I know that I am on the right track.

REFLECTION 18: IMPORTANCE OF THE PLACE OF INFANT MASSAGE IN OUR HEALING FROM PND

My Ayurveda studies and learning about the benefits of *Abhyanga* or massage for the mother using warm oil, led me down the pathway of pursuing learning about the place of infant massage in healing.

I became qualified as a Paediatric Massage Consultant (PMC) and CIMI (Certified Infant Massage Instructor) through the Infant Massage Information Service (IMIS), which is based in Sydney and owned by a passionate and wonderful lady Heidi McLoughlin. These further qualifications allow me to teach the benefits of infant massage to other health professionals, as well as teach mothers how to massage their babies.

What I found so fascinating and resonated with me, was the plethora of biochemical changes that infant massage can bring about to both the baby and mother. It plays such an important role in supporting women with post-natal depression by helping their bonding, attachment and biochemical healing.

The act of massaging an infant can increase oxytocin (the 'love' hormone), serotonin, dopamine and melatonin (regulates sleep) which are *all* vital in the biochemical cascade of PND that occurs.

These changes happen in both the mother doing the massage and the baby receiving it. Most anti-depressants work on increasing serotonin and noradrenaline, and possibly dopamine depending on which medication is chosen. If you are doing massage and these neurotransmitters are increasing in your body naturally, then hopefully this will allow for a faster recovery or medication not being required if you are experiencing only a slight imbalance.

Infant massage also reduces the stress hormone, cortisol, which can play a vital role in reducing anxiety and the 'fight or flight' response. This can already be up-regulated with sleep-deprivation and the effect of the biochemical cocktail that is happening within the body after birth, so it is important to reduce our cortisol in order to reduce our symptoms and to calm our aggravated nervous system.

I also love the enhanced bonding and attachment that is proven to occur with the infant massage, that is so crucial in this early stage. I did the bare minimum with my boys in those early days because I felt so unbelievably disconnected from the whole process. I now wish I had known about the effects it can induce and performed infant massage on them. Maybe then, Ari wouldn't have memories of me being 'sick and dark' and through this massage, my heart-centre may have restored sooner. Touch could well be the best bonding tool available and I shunned it, riddled with my dark and obtrusive thoughts.

Learning the insights, research and clinical trials as to all of the benefits, I also want the world to know about them. I want to teach as many mothers how to massage their babies correctly, especially those suffering with post-natal depression. I hope that it can bring access to the bonding and attachment in such a profound way, so you can walk your way into healing more easily and faster than I did.

We get so caught up in the 'doing' tasks like washing, feeding, cleaning, cooking and tidying that we miss the most magical opportunities to connect and nurture our beautiful babies. In doing massage, we heal ourselves and nourish our biochemistry, whilst creating a bond that is so beautiful and bountiful with our children. I want to shout it from the rooftops as to how simple, yet profound this is and I believe is a very crucial part of the recovery in PND, and to allow the access to this teaching to all mothers.

I would love to see government funding for this teaching to mothers, for its teaching in mother-baby units, in medical schools, pharmacy schools and to all midwives and child health nurses, as to how important this could be in a mother's healing. I am very passionate about this and is a change I would love to see in the near future.

REFLECTION 19: NEED FOR A CONNECTIVE RELATIONSHIP IN PREGNANCY AND CHILDREN VS CLINICAL AND MASCULINE APPROACH

I believe that as a society, when we find out that we are pregnant, we focus so much on the clinical and physical aspects of our baby growing, with our weekly updates of what they look like and how they are developing. Or we focus on doing courses and preparation for the actual birth of the baby, and of course we are busy setting up their nursery and all of the practical aspects of having a baby.

Don't get me wrong, I get it! I did the same! I would send my husband weekly updates on what the boys were doing and what vegetable they looked like at each month! Cute, yes, but not very deeply connective to the process of life that was happening within me!

I enrolled myself as soon as I was pregnant with Kaiyaan into my Hypnobirthing course, as I was adamant I wanted a VBAC and I would do whatever it took to make sure I had one. Yet, what I realise is that there is nothing that we do during our pregnancy to connect with our beautiful baby, the soul connection that we have with each other and the whole spiritual aspect of pregnancy. I made recordings with Kaiyaan towards the end of my pregnancy and wished that I had done it earlier, where I had a primal connection with his soul and connected my whole being to his.

We get so lost in the masculine 'doing' part of pregnancy and so many outcome-based exercises and activities; which all have their place, yes. But what about the divine feminine aspects of motherhood? For all mothers, but especially for first time maidens entering matrescence, where is the encouraging of this connection to the divine feminine within the whole process?

This is where studying Ayurveda truly gave me the heart-centred approach to pregnancy and birthing, that the Western element felt a lot more masculine, scientific and dare I say, very clinical. Ayurveda believes so much in that what a mother takes in through her senses, environment, nutrition, lifestyle, thoughts and emotions, ALL have an impact on the growing baby. Also focusing on energy practices that allow her to feel calm, her *Vata* system (comprised of the air and space elements which are especially stretched during pregnancy and particularly post-birth) to feel the most nourished to soothe her nervous system and are given all of the attention and care that they deserve.

I am in the process of developing more audios, exercises and activities that are things that I wish I did when I was pregnant to become present and connected, rather than focusing on outcome based activities of how I would birth my child or how they are reaching masculine milestones. I want it to be able to help make your pregnancy and post-birth period as bountiful and connected to the divine feminine aspect as possible. To make you as the mother feel so connected to your goddess energy within, that you only can know the divine wisdom and perfection that is within you.

This is in absolute contrast to the *disconnection* that I felt from life but definitely to my children in the depths of my post-natal depression. To experience such disconnection felt *so* heartbreaking to me, that how could I as such a loving mother now, feel this way about my boys? It still riddles my heart with feelings of so much guilt that I could feel anything other than divine connection to the beings that grew inside my body. I now hold them with pure connection and an unconditional love, that came from the acknowledgement of feeling the opposite way. In that sense, perinatal and post-natal depression with the disconnection, is *so* utterly cruel. The cruelest.

You are the creator of this amazing child and are acting as the gatekeeper of them into the world, so we need to revel in this rather than get stuck in the clinical side only. Perhaps harnessing focus on this connection during the throes of perinatal and post-natal depression, may allow us to by-pass the disconnection and almost a 'fake it until you make it' approach, to expedite the journey to reconnect to our children. This is where the learnings of infant massage propelled me into this thinking, and the methodology of creating this connection during a time when we need it the most. By connecting through touch and altering our biochemistry through enhancing oxytocin, serotonin, dopamine, melatonin as well as reducing cortisol, the stress hormone, we can actually allow for a different neural pathway and biochemistry surge to occur within our bodies.

REFLECTION 20: DR SHEFALI'S PORTAL OF PAIN THEORY

Whilst I was in the depth of my depression, my sister introduced me to Dr Shefali who is the most beautiful, heart-felt speaker of the truth and all of her books connect now to me at a soul level... if you have not already delved into her work then I would highly recommend her, once you feel able to of course.

Yet, at the time when she introduced me to the portal of pain concept, I was just not cognitively able to grasp the idea and kept saying that it isn't changing the reality of being IN the portal of pain at the time.

Dr Shefali's premiss is that, it is only through enduring a painful and soul-crushing portal of pain that we can emerge into who we really and truly are. I cannot do justice into how eloquently and beautifully she articulates this concept, so I *implore* you to find her and listen to her speak.

Now as I sit here almost three years since my recovery, I can *only* feel appreciation for the meaning in her message. Now, I can only but *savour* the days. The way the light looks is so different. The way nature looks, smells and sounds to me is so perfect. *All of life* has such a different prospect and outlook to me, that is *completely* transformed from the way I saw it prior to entering this dark hole.

It was through the prospect of leaving it all behind through the intensity of my illness, that has allowed me to remove all the 'stuff' that no longer serves me. To live with an unyielding presence and gratitude for the day that I have today. For the breath that I take today. Had I not been pushed to the ground with *so* much ferocity and been cracked *so badly*, then I would not or could not have re-emerged as the realigned person that I am today.

Whilst you may be feeling that this possibility is so far away or not possible for you, if you are buried deep within the trenches reading this; I promise you that if you keep holding on and walking towards your recovery one step at a time, that you too can experience *all* of this bountiful abundance in life.

It *is* in the rising up after the huge fall where all of the beauty and power lies. You need to hold on, speak out and reach out for the lifeline that you need. The life that *is* amazing and filled with love and connection *is* waiting for you with arms wide open x

REFLECTION 21: AN OPPORTUNITY TO EVOLVE AND SHIFT OUTDATED PARADIGMS UPON HEALING TO LIVE MY BEST LIFE

I had made my recovery 11 weeks post-birth. It took perhaps another two weeks after that to feel fully calibrated and for my biochemistry to be returned back into equilibrium. By Christmas 2018 I was feeling *amazing* and ready to take on the world!

I had realised during my illness that there were underlying mindsets, values, layers that I needed to shift as I felt that they no longer served me. I did not want to live life *any* longer carrying such outdated and heavy baggage. They were simply imprints that had been made throughout my life and imprints can be wiped away. I had the *best* opportunity to start again!

I began a 12-month program of spiritual life coaching with an amazing coach Melissa from Equinox Life Coaching based on the Sunshine Coast. This *absolutely* gave me the most vital learnings, perspectives and healings into my karmic journey and what was happening inside of me, that allowed me to heal *so* many layers from my inner child. I set forth in my life with unbridled enthusiasm and setting down my heavy baggage once and for all.

To the science world this would seem like a lot of 'woo woo', but spirituality has been a huge part of my belief system from as far as I can remember. Understanding karmic ties and spiritual lessons have always been things that I have been interested and passionate about.

I did a lot of inner work into healing my 5-6-year old, that finally gave me so much closure and understanding as to where so many of my inner dialogue and values had set-in. I gained clarity on my purpose. I often asked at various stages 'Why am I here, what is it that I was born to do?'. I always had an inner knowing that there was a purpose and reason why I chose to be born and wondered exactly what I was doing in all of the chapters? Whilst I took on every action with the duty, dedication and commitment that I was brought up with, particularly from my Dad, I always knew there was something amiss and something I didn't quite understand yet.

It was through timeline healing work utilising NLP (Neuro-linguistic programming), that I was able to *finally* break through my value systems and so many layers peeled away like an onion. After each session I felt lighter and more free from carrying outdated thoughts and feelings and I *genuinely* had a new lease on life.

By literally shedding these layers, I was able to connect finally with my true purpose when I stumbled across Ayurveda. Learning this ancient wisdom has resonated so much with me and I would get goose bumps in so many of the classes with my teacher in Perth. I have found that supporting women with their post-natal depression, utilising my Western pharmacist knowledge and my Eastern Ayurveda knowledge together with my paediatric massage training, that I can help bring about change and healing for women to come.

I could never access my 'purpose' through logic and trying to write lists of what I thought they could be! I searched like that for years knowing that my work as a community pharmacist did not truly resonate with what I was born to do and wanted to do for the rest of my life. I *love* the pharmaceutical knowledge and it feels profound, relevant and I love its place in therapy and love being part of the medical industry. However, I felt like I couldn't sustain a lifetime of not evoking *true change* or healing in all those I crossed paths with.

I also feel that in becoming a mother and embracing this divine feminine energy as a creator and nurturer, we have the capacity and ability to facilitate generations of healing within the matriarchal line. My Grandmother was ill with cancer in England when I was going through my PND, and whilst my Mum was with me she was worried about her own Mum. Even when my parents went back to Sydney whilst my in-laws were with us in Perth, they were too scared to go to England in case my situation worsened.

The night I recovered, I had a dream that my Grandmother was speeding behind me coming out of a petrol station in Perth and I remember asking her 'why are you in Perth and why are you tail-gating me?'. She was in transition at that time without a doubt and had come to my dream to say that she was in a hurry. When I had healed, my parents quickly went to England but unfortunately my Grandmother passed away whilst they were in the air. I remember at the moment she passed, though I did not know it until my sister confirmed with me later, but I saw a shadow at our front door. It moved to the next window and then the next window. I knew at that point that it was her, almost checking in on me to make sure that I was OK, and I will always feel her love in that moment. I knew she understood what had happened to me, even though it was never said to her. It was a goodbye and protective gesture to come and see me. I *felt* that ancestral connection and bond in that moment, even though I hardly saw her living in Australia and not being fluent in Hindi or Punjabi, our communication was limited to say the least! Yet, our connection was evident in those encounters and I *knew* that it was deeper than just this life and our souls had seen each other in my darkness and in her transition.

I believe that by healing my inner wounds, I have helped to heal the inner wounds of my mother, her mother and perhaps many other generations past and to come. We are all connected and our healing transcends what we can see, and not just the physical. It has a universal transcendence when we do the inner work and evolve through past conditioning, both culturally and through our experiences and upbringing. This enables us to set forth a new trajectory of our lives and also for our children.

They mirror and watch *all* that we say, do and who we are. Healing our wounds allows us not to sink our clutches and hold onto them and I feel by healing, we can practise conscious living in all aspects. We no longer put accountability and responsibility onto others and *we* reclaim *our* own power.

Perhaps through the journey of life itself we find our inner purpose, our passions and the service that we need to give to others. Perhaps we cannot rush through the chapters, but by being whole and present with each experience, that we can *allow* for the next step to present. One by one, we find our way back home.

During this chapter of your life, even though it may be difficult right now, please know that in time to come you *will* look back and acknowledge your transformation.

Do not give up hope because that time will come. I promise you.

REFLECTION 22: NEED FOR CHANGE AND LIGHT

Another small, yet noteworthy reflection, is one about the importance of needing change. I found that living in places outside of Sydney where there were not clear and distinct seasons, that I needed to have and experience change.

Every day felt like it rolled into the next and the concept of time elapsing and feeling nature change with it, just did not exist. I need to feel the different seasons, the aspect of nature changing to illustrate and give me the feeling that nothing lasts forever. I need the cold of Winter to appreciate the warmth of Summer. Yet, in places where it was only ever a wet or dry season, I felt quite disconnected from the cycle of life, compared to the vast contrast I was used to growing up.

Most people would love continuous blue skies! Therefore, I acknowledge that this is a reflection of my own experience. Yet,

I believe that contrast, change and every season has its place and need for our body, mind and soul. Change allows me to appreciate each season for what it is, and for not needing it to be anything else. It also allows your mind to conceptualise that every season or time in one's life, is not forever and it will evolve as time passes. Nature is wonderful at showing us this. One other reason I am loving being back home in Sydney, is because nature is part of the architecture and landscape here.

I also believe that having light in your home and day is so crucial to your mental health. It has the ability to uplift your mood and is a very powerful tool. After Ari, our apartment was so dark and I can still feel the darkness of my PND when I remember that apartment. Yet, with Kaiyaan we had a big and bright home with a double void and I only remember that space as being bright. I was not so traumatised by my PND in that house, because the light almost washed away all those dark memories there.

If your space is dark, then try opening the blinds and getting fresh air into your place. Go for a walk and feel the sunlight on your skin. Allow it to deeply warm and heal your heart and soul and try to add as much light and life to your home as possible.

Another example of the importance of change would be seen during Covid and the inability to travel. I know that going on holidays and changing the scenery has a huge effect on how we all rejuvenate and refuel. With the lockdowns and inability to freely travel, it has affected the ability to get away and create change into our routine and lifestyle. Change I feel is very therapeutic and breaks the monotony of a very ordered way of life. Since we cannot change the reality of Covid whilst it is here, I would say to add change into your days as much as you can and in whatever ways you can. This will hopefully break the circuit and add elements of variety and spice to your life!

REFLECTION 23: LISTENING TO YOUR INTUITION; YOUR INNER GUIDANCE SYSTEM

I believe in the importance of trusting one's gut intuition, if it is something that you are aware of.

I remember with Kaiyaan in the hospital when the nurse was giving me Motilium, the medication to enhance my breastmilk supply, something told me not to take it just yet and to wait and see how my journey unfolded. It works by enhancing Prolactin, which in turn blocks dopamine as a way to enhance milk production. Upon reflection, I feel that this could have been what sent me into a deeper and more intense depression with him, given that dopamine is a 'feel-good hormone'.

For some reason as the nurse was leaving the room, I stopped her and changed my mind. I had the intuition and I ignored it. To my detriment. So I do believe that if you have an inkling of your intuition, then certainly take heed of it.

We have used our intuition in all of the business and life decisions that we have made. We say yes to things or people if they feel right for us, or we say no or can walk away from decisions if we do not feel they are right for us. This has allowed us to say YES to life, and the journey has been one of transformation! If you live life with complete trust, surrender and faith whilst following your inner guidance system, then you can never look back in regret. Rather it allows you to live a life full of opportunity, action and hope instead of stagnation and an inability to make decisions.

REFLECTION 24: FINAL WORD

This final reflection is more of a 'final word' of what I would love to advocate for and see moving forward. It would be amazing for women not to suffer in silence or greater than necessary in generations to come; possibly my daughters-in-law or nieces and even their children.

Moving forward I want to see, partake of and rally for more clinical trials into concrete quantifiable causes. It is essential to know solid and definite underlying reasons as to what may predispose women into getting PNDA. It will allow for management to rebalance and restore such discrepancies prior to embarking upon pregnancy, before any more people lose their lives, or cause families to break down. Without knowing key fundamental causes, how can we ever see change and progress in this area? We need to move forward with a greater understanding and clarity as to what nutritional or biochemical imbalances can be restored before, during or after pregnancy, to help support these mothers.

My wish is that I can go into a Mothers and Baby unit and while video recording, interview midwives, nurses, and other mothers that have been through these units, to show women what that road may look like. I feel that it is important to allay any fears surrounding the services. I want to provide reassurance as to what happens there, and alleviate any concerns that their babies will be taken away.

It may be a very healing process for me to undertake this exercise, as I was filled with apprehension about this. I hope that by shining the light on practical and available services, that we can pave the way for a journey to recovery, rather than live crippled with doubt and fear. Education is the way out of this darkness. Shining a light on what we can offer, as well as making more services available, is a vital step to take.

I definitely would love to see more funding and support tools surrounding babies and sleep. Not having adequate sleep will not encourage your body and mind to heal, given that sleep deprivation is a well-known torture tactic! The saying of 'sleep when the baby sleeps' is also not helpful, when they only nap for 40 minutes and/or your baby is waking 7 to 8 times a night. Coupled with not sleeping at all for the first 11 weeks except a few hours here or there, I had severe sleep deprivation and sleep debt that took a long time to restore. When 6 months rolled around I was beyond ready to start sleep training them, and was so grateful that they took to it so well. I have not looked back at all. I know that for a lot of women embarking upon an exercise like this, can aggravate their anxiety. Leaving their children alone to navigate through finding ways to sleep, can be very overwhelming and can feel utterly heartless. I totally appreciate that and this is not written to enhance your feelings of overwhelm!

However, I knew that I could not sustain this poor level of sleep and knew that everyone would be better equipped to handle the day and get the most from our time together, if we were all rested. I know there are sleep training services such as Tresillian and Karitane, which can be so helpful. Different States have different services available and you will need to chat with your doctor about the best option for you to get a referral. I believe that access and availability needs to be all around Australia, and other options available if the mother is unable to stay there with her illness. If sleep is an ongoing issue, then do chat with your partner and see what options are available that you are both comfortable with. Share the journey of restoring sleep in your home together. This is a priority, but should not cause you to feel overwhelmed by the whole process. I simply know that having uninterrupted sleep throughout our home, benefitted each and every one of us.

I would love funding for childcare to be reassessed, so that all women have access to subsidised child care. This is in order to allow them to remain current in the work force with up-to-date experience. It is important that women and families do not crunch the numbers as to whether it is 'viable' to go to work, subtracting the full cost of child care; as they cannot add unquantifiable figures of value like their identity, ability to earn an income and have their own financial credibility and power to this equation. Their financial control should never be lost, in case somewhere down the track a separation from their partner occurs. They need help to re-enter the workplace as their skills may be out-of-date, due to lack of current experience and participation. This adds a further burden on the mother. This could be a contribution to domestic control or abuse, where there can be a financial power play and control aspect here. Equality is paramount.

Following from this topic, another point of possible contention and yet one that I feel the need to voice, is the disparity in Australia between the private versus public sector in healthcare. I feel like I was able to be seen quickly because my OB was able to get me in to the psychologist, and the practice I went to was affordable to me with respect to the out-of-pocket costs. What if I could not though?

It makes me wonder what happens to patients who are waiting to gain medical treatment and what they do in the meantime. What happens if you cannot afford the gap payment? Do these women get lost in the system and pretend like they are coping, when in fact they are in dire need of help and attention?

I would strongly advocate for Telehealth appointments to be available for psychiatrists and psychologists to be continuous and world-wide. This is so that no one slips through the system because they are so unwell to make logistics work. People need to understand that even getting out of bed and dressed, seems like such a mammoth task. I can see how people do decide they cannot go on, as it all seems and FEELS unbelievably upstream. Whilst I can fully understand that non-verbal cues, feeling the energy and emotion of a patient is more easily done in a face-to-face setting, I also personally have felt the logistic and energetic struggle to simply attend an appointment. With Ari in Cairns I remember finishing my appointment, putting him in the capsule in the car. I then sat on the front seat and just cried until I had no more tears to cry. It was as if it took all of my energy just to get there and through that appointment.

I would love to see FTA (Failure to Attend) statistics for these face-to-face appointments and compare these to Telehealth appointments in the same category, and then use this data to see whether there is a benefit in keeping scheduled appointments. Unlike a non-urgent dental appointment, an FTA in this setting could be a matter of someone taking their own life or not, so it is crucial.

I would advocate strongly for teaching the benefits of infant massage, and teach all of the health care professionals and mothers around the world about this modality. All medical practitioners, midwives, child health nurses and pharmacists who are in the forefront of maternal and infant care, need to be trained in the benefits and place of infant massage. My hope is that it forms the foundation of all antenatal education to set them forward with the best skills possible to nurture and nourish their connection with their children.

I would love for families within the community to see a new mother as a beautiful divine feminine embodiment that they can be of service to. If they can arrange a meal delivery service amongst a few families, arrange for groceries, help with school drop off/collection if needed, it can ease some of the burden on new families. This is even more crucial for those people that have no family support nearby. If we can become more 'tribal' in support, then our mothers will feel like she is being held in the most nurturing and organic way. This is especially true if the help is not intrusive, almost invisible where she does not have to arrange logistics herself or return things, and can simply focus on resting, healing and looking after her body, mind, spirit and baby.

Another profoundly strong feeling that I have not been able to shake, is towards all of those mothers who may be suffering from post-natal depression and could potentially be adding the strain of a chronic and seriously ill baby or child, a physical illness, financial stress and/or domestic abuse. How can one endure all of this together? I know that I stand in a very privileged position and the reality of suffering beyond just PND, *absolutely* breaks my heart. I would hope that the universe isn't that cruel as to give anyone more than one turbulent and stressful situation at a time; but this is idealism at its finest.

Yet, for these women that have the world of struggle on their shoulders, I would hope that they have the best amount of support around them to help get through this time, in addition to seeking treatment for themselves. However, if their families are not living close by and with Covid, my heart goes out to those women who are so utterly helpless. I hope that as a society we can check in on *all* the mothers all around the world, and see how we can be of service to them. Helping even one woman through a treacherous time, is truly being purposeful and making the world a place with more love and kindness.

After Ari was born we had his horoscope made in Sri Lanka, more out of cultural habits and my own personal interest in astrology and numerology. The horoscope had written that Ari's Mum would be very sick when he was born, because it took all of her energy to bring him into the world.

Yet, it got me wondering what power and strength my boys hold to have caused such an energetic sapping away of my energy. Truth be told I would endure any of this pain again and again for their presence here on this Earth, and it brings me a real solace in thinking that they potentially carry such a strong energy field and this is the sacrifice that I had to make to bring these beautiful souls into the world. Whether it is true, only time will tell, but with their great names chosen, Ari meaning 'the Lion God and the one who is on the right direction', Kaiyaan meaning 'the universe' and Mahanama meaning 'The Great name', I hope this sets their future true to their names given...no pressure, right?!

Funnily enough when Chandi and I got married, we had our horoscope read and it said that we would have two children. At the time since we both come from a family of three children, we always planned to have three and thought the horoscope was wrong. Suffice to say that after the experience of having our two beautiful boys, Chandi has had a vasectomy and it was my Christmas present to him! I had been recovered for a good 2 to 3 weeks at that point, and I vowed that we could not endure this one more time, so off I sent him to the snip snip doctor!

I went to my GP before moving to Sydney and happened to ask about what options were available to me. She giggled saying that unless I was planning to cheat on my husband, there is no need for both of us to be operated on so to just relax. I have giggled about that many times since!

The irony is that though we have worked so much on our healing, things pop up in often the most unlikely of scenarios and life situations. We have made peace with the fact that our family is complete and we want to help others navigate their way through this journey, but feel like we could not test the fates of the universe again.

Our family is complete and what a journey our beautiful boys have taken us on with their arrival x

CHAPTER 3

MINDSETS

A nother important area that during my post-natal depression I was privy to identify and observe were certain mindset traits and characteristics. I was able to catch myself having certain inner dialogues and assessments of certain situations, which ordinarily occur on auto-pilot. Yet, during the process of healing as well as my twelve month coaching program, it allowed me to question certain thought processes. It became easier to identify what mindsets were serving me and what was holding me back.

During the thick of being in post-natal depression, it may not necessarily be the best time to unveil and dive into analysing one's mindset without working with a trained professional. Any element of adding criticism or judgement to our patterns may hinder our ability to recover. I believe that whilst awareness can be a good thing, if you are becoming judgemental about what you are observing, then there is no critical urgency in observing your patterns until you are feeling better biochemically. No doubt you have had these patterns for many years so waiting another month or two, or however long it may take, is not going to make or break you. These observations are simply ones that I was able to identify during my process, that I feel pertinent to share.

It is not often that we have someone to be our sounding board and reflect on whether the way in which we view circumstances and life is conducive to our growth, or whether it is holding us back. It very much is a choice that we have at each and every juncture, whether we choose thoughts and a mindset that is expansive or progressive and one for our highest growth and evolution. Or we can choose to be restrictive, limited and very constricted in our mindset. Both polarities have very visceral feelings behind them and they do give rise to energy and an effect at a cellular level each time we make a choice of thought.

Think as an example the situation where your car breaks down. Imagine that as a reaction or emotion you choose anger, frustration, 'why does this always happen to me?' type thinking. By choosing to respond with anger to this situation, every cell of your being, your energy field, those people around you in that energy field and the environment will be subjected to this harsh, volatile and all-encompassing emotion. Anger has been associated in the Eastern modality to be connected to our liver and adrenergic systems, and this energy that ensues can then impact our bodily systems.

Now, think of the same scenario but this time responding in a more flexible and expansive way. Being in solution-mode, calm, centred, not taking it personally and using your energy into getting the situation resolved. Your emotions are calm, the people in the car with you feel calm, your energy field and the environment has not changed in frequency because of your emanating emotions. You are able to call NRMA or RAC quickly and you move along with your day seamlessly, as if nothing but a minor inconvenience popped up.

On one hand, it may seem easier said than done. On another hand, you may think that of course you would respond in the second way and yet, in reality you may actually respond in the first way! By being mindful of checking-in on how you view and see the world, you can adjust the filter of your glasses (not your Instagram camera!) to make more conscious and mindful choices in thoughts. It will always feel less energetically straining, more easy and effortless to make expansive and growth mindset thoughts. Through conscious living you can change the trajectory of your thought train into one that is serving you and taking you to the right station, with all the thoughts and reactions that you make. It is never too late to make the shift and just like a muscle, the more you practise it, the stronger and more natural it will become.

Don't get me wrong, with two young boys I am often losing my patience and responding with frustration when they do not listen or are fighting...somehow always when I am on the phone?! Yet, I am able to check in, take a breath and re-set myself when I can feel my internal system responding in a non-conducive way. I believe that we are always a work in progress and we have never 'arrived' to perfection or a static way of being. I often utilise some *Pranayama/* breathing techniques to best support my nervous system. I am human and I am fallible, so work always needs to be done as our situation and stimuli constantly change. Yet, I approach it in a loving and compassionate way rather than criticism. I am proud that I can identify my areas to improve and take action steps towards shifting what is not serving me.

I had a limiting thought mindset and had a lot of layers that I needed to first identify and then catch myself doing, so that I could make conscious changes for my self-betterment. It is not playing a blame game on oneself and using it as a way to be critical and unkind to yourself. It is however, a great way to be the observer as to HOW you perceive life and make one step forward to a more expansive way of thinking and being.

I have listed below several very limiting, restrictive and constricted thought processes and mindsets, that I could definitely reflect on once I had recovered from my post-natal depression. Whilst I did not imbibe all of them, I have listed what else I thought may hinder our filter when viewing life. Some of these reflections may be repetitions from previous ones, but I felt that they pertained to mindset specifically so have included them in here.

These thoughts could not come during my PND if they were not seeds deeply lodged somewhere in my subconscious, thoughts or belief system to begin with. When you squeeze or squash an orange then only orange juice can come out because that is what is inside. In the same way that such negative and sometimes harmful ways of thinking can only present and come out, if they are already planted deep within. It then required a lot of inner reflection and work with some amazing Earth angels to strip away many limiting thought processes and belief systems.

We all have shadows, which is what it means to be alive and human. Even a flower has a shadow when light is shined behind it. We shine our light on the aspects that we want to heal but not in a self-deprecating way, rather with gratitude for allowing them to serve the purpose they needed to and then letting them go with the new found awareness of no longer needing them.

I am constantly listening to podcasts, reading new books, going to sound healings and enrolling in courses for my internal growth, much to my husband's horror! Yet, I feel like if we are not perpetually evolving, then being stagnant is just a monumental waste of time being here on planet Earth. We have bountiful and endless opportunities to live our best life always and it is so liberating to be able to embrace all of it now with my health reinstated.

SUMMARY OF RESTRICTIVE THOUGHTS AND MINDSETS

1. Perfectionism
2. All or nothing
3. Catastrophising, over generalising, jumping to conclusions
4. Negative lens, pessimistic

5. The 'grass is greener' mentality
6. Black and white mentality
7. 'Could have, should have' thinking
8. Control
9. Organised, structured, routine
10. Comparison
11. Masculine mindset vs divine feminine
12. Victim mentality
13. Self-blame
14. Perceiving life as a dress rehearsal vs being present
15. Rigid and needing to study/prepare
16. Fortune telling
17. Fear

WHAT ARE SOME LIMITING AND RESTRICTIVE THOUGHTS AND MINDSETS?

1. PERFECTIONISM
The internal need for everything to be *perfect* or it is just not good enough. Holding this standard for yourself and also onto others. This can make it feel like you are never satisfied or that nothing is good enough, unless it is exactly how you want it to be or look like.

The irony is that life is never perfect. There are so many variables that can present at any time, so waiting for situations to be 'perfect' is not realistic. Parenthood throws the ability of perfectionism out the window because we cannot control every aspect of our children, their health, their behaviours and personalities. Wanting it to look or be a certain way is idealistic and not something that can actually occur. At least in my renewed perspective!

2. ALL OR NOTHING
Working tirelessly for days on end until the task was complete and then crash and burn at the end, was how things looked to me. Or on the polar extreme, I would do nothing at all because of the fear of

failure or not doing it well enough! It is a very *Vata and Pitta dosha* characteristic within me in an Ayurvedic perspective, but I know that this extreme mindset cannot serve anyone well.

Balance is the key for sustainable success and longevity. Burning the midnight oil every day then sleeping for a month is not practical with children. Taking bite sized pieces, chewing and then assimilating is ideal. This would look like working then resting at a manageable pace until the job is complete.

3. CATASTROPHISING, OVER-GENERALISING, JUMPING TO CONCLUSIONS

This is making very grandiose statements like 'nothing ever goes right for me' or 'things like this always happen to me'. It does not leave room for anything in between and are very extreme ways to think.

For that example, with the car breaking down, a catastrophic response of 'this always happens to me!' would fill your body with cortisol, the stress hormone and take you to a heightened state of arousal and very much into victim mode. Comparing this to responding with calm and resolve, would fill your body with a very different feeling and allow you to make clear decisions without judgement.

4. NEGATIVE LENS/ PESSIMISTIC

My continuous loop during my PND was described as 'very muddy and sticky thoughts'. Always viewing things as negative, hard and upstream rather than being flexible, go with the ebb and flow. These opposite descriptions have very different feelings associated with them when you hear and imagine the words within your body.

5. THE 'GRASS IS GREENER' MENTALITY

The idea that other people have it easier than you or even that life was easier 'back then' or will become easier or better 'if x, y, or z happens'. This is taking away one's own personal power of watering our own grass and feeding it to grow.

It is also important to remember that not everything you see is as it seems. The story of us going for a walk as a family looking picture perfect from the outside, yet the reality was an absolute mess beyond what anyone could have imagined upon first glance. What may seem to be better or easier does not change the reality of where you are.

Whilst it is great to have goals or aspirations, the grass is green where you water it.

6. BLACK AND WHITE MENTALITY
This is similar to the all or nothing mindset. I had a very rigid and stubborn view on the way things had to be and turn out and if it didn't look that way, then I would feel like it was a failure. The way I birthed my babies and whether I could breastfeed definitely had this black and white perspective on the way I viewed it. If my body did not do what I wanted it to do, then I viewed it as a fail rather than celebrate the glorious achievements in between.

Life however, is not black and white but has various shades of grey and so much beautiful colour! If we only stick with these monotones and the very rigid views of how we want things to be, then we will miss the beauty in all the shades that lie in between. Sometimes the outcome will be far better than what we could even imagine, if we only allow ourselves to experience and value it.

7. 'COULD HAVE, SHOULD HAVE' THINKING
This hindsight way of living, is looking in the past in the hope that the outcomes could change; however, there is no way to change the past. A significant amount of energy is wasted in worrying about what you could have done differently, because the outcome can never be altered. We need to accept that we made certain choices

with the knowledge that we had at that time, and that is all we can expect from ourselves or others.

We can only learn from our decisions and amend what our choices may be moving forward, if we are presented with the same crossroad again. We cannot however, change the past so there is no need to live life looking in the rear-view mirror. This can only make us place blame, not feel satisfied with the choices that we did make and since the outcome cannot be altered, then what a waste of precious energy and time.

8. CONTROL

This aspect in parenting has been a hard one to let go of, yet is a very important one! Firstly, I cannot control what my children do, how they behave every moment or what they will say. It is actually exhausting trying to control every aspect of what they do and in the end I feel like I am the Queen of nagging. It is also not allowing them to be who they truly are and they are all here to live out their destiny.

I feel like it is a very restrictive and stifling way to live life, in that it does not allow the freedom of life to unfold in a possibly better way than one could even imagine. We can only have control, based on what we know to be right or true. Life can expand our mind and knowledge of all aspects if we simply *allow* and go with the flow. In this way, our awareness expands rather than being stuck in wanting it a certain way.

The feelings around trying to control a particular situation compared to going with the flow and allowing what organically will transpire, have two very different feelings and handle on them. One feels constrictive and the other feels like freedom.

9. ORGANISED, STRUCTURED, ROUTINED

Having a baby turns this capability upside down on its head! I have a *Vata dosha* composition, which is comprised of air and space. This means that I thrive on grounding and solidifying aspects of routine and predictability.

Therefore, I struggled with the erratic sleeping, eating, mess and chaos that comes with children, especially in the early newborn stage. I had to let that rigid need go to some extent, otherwise I would be living with a very dissatisfied perspective of the world throughout my entire journey of motherhood, which would be for a long time!

I have found ways in attaining the feeling of grounding with other strategies as well as grasp onto what routine I can, in order to have that same effect; though not as rigid and strict as before. However, the acknowledgment that structure is not realistic all the time has given me a lot more peace given the reality of having children, and I have become a lot more OK with the fluidity of the new 'normal'.

10. COMPARISON

I have always lived with wishing I was a fly on the wall so I could see what others did or how they lived! Chandi has never understood this and concentrates on which lane he is driving in. I have seen the way he lives (and drives!) serves him, and I can also see how I am riddled with worrying about others, that it affects how I live…and drive! It is the 'people pleasing' aspect of myself that cares so much about others and puts my own needs or wants aside so as not to disappoint anyone else, even if it is to my own detriment.

However, when it comes to comparison it either stems from a superiority complex of thinking you are better than someone or something, or from an inferiority complex, which is where you feel 'less than'. Either way, there is judgement involved in the way you view others and yourself. We were taught this concept from a young age reading the 'Bhagavad Gita', which is a sacred Indian text. Life needs more compassion, empathy and understanding and less judgement, and this pertains to the way we view and look at ourselves too.

I would highly recommend Melissa Ambrosini's book *'Comparisonitis'* which talks all about this 'toxic' trait and how we need to stop comparing ourselves to others. It is an easy and great read if you get a chance that has lots of strategies to help pull oneself away from this trait.

11. MASCULINE MINDSET VS DIVINE FEMININE

I looked at facts, the science, the logic and not intuition or connection during my pregnancy and definitely during my post-natal experience. I needed to honour my inner wisdom and the trust in being able to nurture and care for my children, as there was no one else who could do a better job. However, the disruption in my biochemistry caused me to completely lose trust in myself, have low self-esteem and low confidence, which made me feel like a duck out of water.

Yet, the divine feminine is *so* connected to a mother's heart-centre, so in tune with her own inner guidance system and nurtures herself and all those around her. The biochemical warfare within me switched off my capacity to feel. Yet, I wonder if it was because I was already starting from the baseline of harnessing the divine masculine within me more than my divine feminine, that this is what presented when I was squashed like an orange?

12. VICTIM MENTALITY

I felt very resentful towards my body as to how and why it could betray me like this. I felt like I was the only one experiencing this so no one could understand and I felt like it was just not fair. The 'why me?' mindset. Unfortunately, having this type of thinking does not change the outcome and ends up making you feel more frustrated, resentful and upset about the situation.

Although, I would not have understood or agreed to this at the time; but the reality is, everything in life whether it be good or bad happens for us and not to us. It is for our growth and higher evolution that we are presented certain challenges.

If you are in the thick of a deep post-natal depression, you can throw the book at me now! I get it! It is so hard to rationalise any suffering as being beneficial when you are going through it and to sugar coat it in the form of spiritual evolution.

Yet, I want you to keep faith that you will look back and you *will* get through this time, and be grateful for certain insights that may happen, as long as you allow space for your healing and recovery. Just let go of this victim mindset after you have gone through the process of letting out your anger and frustration about the situation...You've got this!

13. SELF-BLAME
This is a very toxic trait and I especially did it for things I didn't know. Yet, how could I know what I didn't know? It holds feelings opposite to forgiveness and self-compassion, and is being very harsh on oneself.

We are our own worst critics. Yet, we need to start treating ourselves, our feelings, our decisions and everything in between in the same way that we would talk to or treat our children or best friend. We would cheer them on and not let them speak about themselves that way. We would hold onto all the beautiful things they do and are. We need to do more of this for ourselves.

I blamed myself for the way I birthed Ari, not being able to breast-feed, for having PND and not being prepared for it. These are all *limiting* thoughts and very similar to the 'should have, could have' thoughts that live in the past and does not change the current reality, so it is a monumental waste of energy and time!

14. PERCEIVING LIFE AS A DRESS REHEARSAL VS BEING PRESENT

I realised that I had this trait reflecting upon spending years working in a job that did not light up my soul with joy. I constantly would think that life would be better later or become 'ideal' soon. I was missing the present and wishing my days away for an imaginary future that may never roll on by.

Life is for living right now; not tomorrow or next year or when this or that happens. It is *right now* with the current breath that we take. It was only from feeling happy to reaching the depths of rock bottom and wanting to leave it all behind overnight, that turned this perspective completely on its head for me.

Whilst it is wonderful to have goals and aspirations, I realised that tomorrow or even later in the day is not promised, so to not wait until things get better to truly live because that time may *never* come. By speaking up and stepping into your recovery, it will allow for you to live your amazing life also right here and now.

I am blessed that my post-natal depression taught me this, as well as being blessed with my boys. I might sometimes crave the noise, mess, fighting and chaos to move onto the next phase, yet I realise in the times that I am not paying attention that I am missing them being so perfect and cute right now! I catch myself and then return to savouring every conversation, every laugh, things we see and do together with *all* of my being. They teach me how to be right here in the moment and their forgiveness also teaches me how amazing it is to dust yourself off and rise up for the next adventure.

They are my biggest teachers and for that I am truly humbled.

15. RIGID AND NEEDING TO STUDY/PREPARE

I am an excellent student in general where I can learn something and then be able to put it into practice with relative ease and grace...

and clearly very humble! Yet, after having a wonderful pregnancy and delivering this baby, there was no manual at the end that came with him from the sky and I absolutely felt like a duck out of water!

It was as if delivering the baby was the exam and then I was thrown a million other exams, that I had not studied for and felt *very* overwhelmed! I was annoyed that no one 'taught' or prepared me for it and annoyed at myself for not reading about it. Yet, how could I know what I didn't know? It was very much a 'learn as you go' mentality now instead of my usual read, study and *do* which is a very Type A personality type and very masculine. It does connect with the control, stubborn and rigid mindsets compared to going with the flow, being flexible and the 'don't sweat the small stuff' mindsets!

Thankfully, in time I have learned to be more discerning as to what requires my attention and what is just kids being kids and to ride the wave. Perhaps that is what time and experience with children has brought, and it is refreshing to know that all of these mindsets can be changed and nothing is 'forever' or too late to change. It just requires an awareness of what is serving you and then deciding on whether you are willing to let it go.

16. FORTUNE TELLING
This is predicting a dark and pessimistic view of the future. This parallels to the catastrophising and over-generalising type of thinking. It is seeing the cup as half empty and assuming life is hard work and will not go the way you want it to.

Ironically, if one has this thought process, most likely scenarios will present to support your premiss, unless you are mindfully aware of what is happening. The concept of where energy flows, intention goes and grows. Ideally it would be good to drop the doom and gloom future projections, as this will continuously beat down your soul and add to the feelings of helplessness and the road to recovery looking far away or not possible. This type of thinking cannot best serve your recovery and healing.

17. FEAR

This is a *big one* and includes; the fear of judgement, fear of the baby being taken away, a fear of being seen as unwell, a fear of everything going wrong instead of right, and a fear of this being your reality forever.

I was too scared to go to the mothers' groups because I thought everyone would be able to see how unwell I was. I was scared to see people who knew me because immediately they would know that something was wrong.

Fear is what kept me *stuck* in silence for so long. Fear is also a crippling part of anxiety and can riddle one's mind with *so* many thoughts of what may occur when in reality the odds are very low. Fear is the opposite to love and feels very constrictive in nature, instead of expansive and liberating.

FINAL WORD ON MINDSETS

These mindsets may serve purpose in many circumstances and there is no 'right or wrong' way to think. It is important to notice what your thought patterns are, where they stem from and what purpose within you and your life that they serve.

Is it to protect yourself and the possibility of being disappointed? Is it for self-preservation and protecting yourself from getting hurt or being wrong? There is no judgment, only an *opportunity* for observation, reflection and a choice as to where you wish to direct your thoughts, based on what you feel is serving you and what you feel may serve you better.

If you imagine within your body how these words below *feel* when you think of them, as a way to illustrate the difference between very limited and constrictive thoughts vs expansive and growth-centred thoughts;

Jealousy vs Compassion
Fear Vs Love
Hate vs Kindness
Resentment vs Forgiveness
Hostility vs Empathy

I would recommend that if you observe your thought processes, then work through your mindset with a psychologist or trained professional. They are experts in the field of getting to the root cause and helping you to identify *where* limiting thought processes may be coming from and taking you in life; the decisions that you make and the way in which you perceive the world. Whilst in the depths of your post-natal depression this may not necessarily be the first priority, however it is something to work through with them as a way to shift your inner mindset. They can provide you with relevant coping mechanisms as strategies to help you live your *best* life, without anything unnecessary altering your lenses.

I have done a lot of work to change my victim mentality of things happening 'to' me to one of things happen 'for' me. I have looked for compassion, empathy, kindness, forgiveness and use open communication as a way to remove any residual resentment and pain. I continue to shed layers of myself that no longer serve me and we are so fortunate that we have access to so many coaches, psychologists, personal trainers just to name a few, that can help to shift the way in which we perceive things.

I love listening to podcasts whilst I am walking or driving as a way to constantly expand my perspective and knowledge. I love listening to Jay Shetty who is a very inspirational speaker and has written a brilliant book called *'Think like a Monk'.* It has provided me with countless tools and practical tips into realigning my mindsets and the way in which I choose to view the world. I would highly recommend him whilst you are driving to work, going for a walk or are cooking. His work is very inspiring and transformative.

Find people who you resonate with when you feel ready and able, that you feel take you to a better place each time you listen or read their content. It is a great way to gain a fresh perspective on the way we view and take to life.

No guilt or feeling critical over any observations you make. There is only opportunity for breakthroughs.

HEALTH TIP:

WHAT BOOKS, PODCASTS OR INFLUENCERS DO I RESONATE WITH?

+ Everything by Dr Shefali Tsabary

+ Everything by Jay Shetty

+ The Melissa Ambrosini Show Podcast

+ Oprah's Super Soul Podcast

+ Everything by Gabby Bernstein

+ Everything by Eckhart Tolle

+ Pregnancy with Physio Laura Podcast

+ The Postnatal Depletion Cure by Dr Oscar Serrallach

+ Untethered Soul by Michael A. Singer

+ You are abundant by Belinda Grace

+ You can heal your life by Louise Hay

+ Dr Joe Dispenza

+ The Highest Self Podcast with Sahara Rose

+ Deepak Chopra with his meditations and Ayurveda knowledge

+ Radhi Devlukia-Shetty

+ Wayne Dyer

+ Robin Sharma

+ Tony Robbins

+ Audible is great if you are finding it hard to focus and read a physical book

+ Following positive influencers on Facebook and Instagram is also feeding me positive stories and I unfollow anything that creates negativity or feelings that I recognise that do not serve my highest good. Everything we take in through our senses have an influence on how we think and feel, so be discerning with what you consume through all of your 5 senses

Disclaimer: I did not have the ability to read these books when I was unwell. If you find this overwhelming, just keep these resources in your tool kit for when you do feel ready to delve into them. There is no pressure to do and read everything as you recover. Take it nice and steady!

CHAPTER 4

SELF-TALK

The way in which we speak to ourselves through our own inner dialogue can be either positive and constructive, or negative and self-defeating. Whilst it does tie in together with the concept of thoughts and mindset that was discussed in chapter 3, I believe it also includes our tone and the WAY in which we speak internally to our self.

These patterns can be imprinted at a very young age during our formative years and may stem from the way someone, a teacher or our parents spoke to us. We often carry this forward in the way in which we talk and treat ourselves. This can absolutely shape how we have this inner monologue or dialogue internally, and has the ability to last a lifetime.

It is also an important process to observe and reflect upon the way in which we do speak to ourselves and to change the tone, words and theme from a hostile or negative approach, to one of kindness and compassion. The way in which we feel internally at a cellular level as a result, will change remarkably for the positive.

I believe that no one would yell or scream at a child to make them feel bad intentionally to crush them. Yet, perhaps that is where it stemmed from within us and we have carried it forward through our adolescence and now adulthood. Who is it serving? How can it be conducive to our health and well-being? How can it be supporting our feelings towards self-love and a healthy interaction with our body, mind and spirit? We would not speak to a stranger or a friend the way we sometimes can speak to ourselves. I do not want to generalise as I know that not everyone has a critical inner self-dialogue, and potentially this could be an individual trait vs a universal trait.

My amazing psychologist during my first visit, where I was stuck in my repetitive loop that was caused by my biochemical imbalance, gave me a copy of this diagram below. It was an excellent illustration as to what occurs with this loop and how talking more about the loop, in fact strengthens it and consolidates it even more.

My Aunty had therefore instructed to cut me off whenever I was going on my tangent and to bring me back into reality, in order to change the trajectory of my thoughts. Though I did not understand it at the time, the science behind redirecting my thoughts to more constructive and positive ones was for my overall recovery and enabling me to come out of this ongoing vicious cycle that was our reality.

A shortened summary illustration is below:

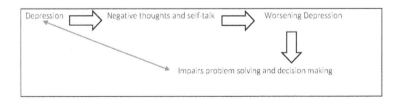

It is through the negative thoughts and self-talk that can consolidate and strengthen our loop and depression. It is therefore important to be observant as to what your inner conversation is within and then to make mindful and concerted efforts to redirect those thoughts.

I have been an advocate throughout as to the effect of thoughts and emotions and their impact on our body at a cellular level. Imagine if we have one person who tells themselves 'you can do it, you are bountiful and can achieve anything you put your mind to'. Then there is the other person who says 'you always get things wrong, you never get anything right, why do I even bother?'. The internal effect within the bodies of these two very opposite tonal conversations, will be *entirely* different.

I recommend if you have not already done so, to follow the work of Masaru Emoto and his experiment on the effects of different words, emotions and energies and the impact that it makes on the structure of water molecules. He illustrates the profound effect on the shape and structure of water molecules. When the water is infused with love and gratitude it looks so different to 'I hate you'. 'I can do it' looks so different to 'I can't do it' as well as 'peace vs war' as some examples.

This experiment illustrates the visceral differences at a molecular level when we speak to water and how it can look. Considering that we are made up of approximately 70 percent of water in some areas of our body, there is *no* doubt that the way in which we speak to ourselves has an impact at a very cellular and molecular level.

Another experiment that he did was placing a grain of rice in a glass of water. The power that different emotions of 'love, hate, thank you, prayer' can have to the consistency and how the water and rice look, is another very visual example as to the power that is held in words and emotions.

Imagine speaking to ourselves as we would to our children, with the intention and essence of nurturing, honouring them so that they can thrive and not just survive. If we choose compassion, kindness, love and forgiveness instead of being critical, judgemental, self-blaming or hateful then imagine the difference in imprint at a cellular level within our bodies?

We are also the best example as to how our children talk to themselves as they watch and mirror all that they see. Sometimes it is not what we teach them but what they absorb through watching and imitating us. If we speak to ourselves showing self-respect, responsibility, kindness and compassion, then this is the tone they will take with themselves. They will in turn take this tone to their friends, which has a rippling effect throughout the world for generations to come. We hold *that* much power when we reclaim back our power and responsibility, to treat ourselves with the respect that we deserve.

It also parallels to the principle in Ayurveda, *Pragya Aparadha* which is this loss of knowingness of our intellect or no longer remembering that we are the divine. If we know the true essence that is within us, then how *could* we speak to ourselves with anything other than love and compassion? It has been the re-learning of this state that has allowed my heart to expand and widen. It also allows my mind to broaden and grow and for me to feel more connected to my soul than ever before. All is not lost and there is no such thing as being too late.

We can change the direction of our self-talk at any point and there is no time better than now x

CHAPTER 5

HORMONE CHANGES

I have always been very 'temperamental' as my Dad would say leading up to my cycle from an early age. Without fail, five to six days prior to my cycle, I am super cranky and very moody. Much to the despair of all four boys around me!

I started my cycle relatively early and wonder if it had anything to do with the foods I was eating, as I was quite chubby. What came first? I wonder if the chemicals, stressors or environment sent me into an early adolescence and whether, if I was more mindful about choices of the 'pollutants', that I put into my system, that it would have altered its onset.

I have been examined in the last few months with extensive blood tests which showed that I have oestrogen dominance. My Integrative GP recommended that I cull as many environmental pollutants from skincare, deodorants, plastics and the type of water I drink as they all can affect this balance.

I was very confused as to what had caused my PND until I saw my doctor at The Elizabeth Clinic in Perth. She explained it to me in very simple terms that gave me such a profound sense of peace and understanding. She explained to me that our hormone levels drop from pregnancy to breastfeeding *100 times* in level and this is a very large and significant drop. This happened to me at day 5 on both occasions when my milk had come-in. This change-over in hormones within my body, flicked a switch in my brain that derailed my thoughts off the track and sent me on my hideous loop. The doctor felt that this was caused by the hormonal drop, which then triggered a huge biochemical cascade to occur.

There was no way that the switch could be flicked back without balancing the distorted biochemistry. There was also no way of healing my thoughts and body, without establishing balance and harmony within my neurotransmitters of dopamine, serotonin and noradrenaline. To be fair, once the biochemistry was corrected I immediately felt amazing and the work needed to shift my thoughts was not too difficult. Once I had obtained my homeostasis, I was able to have the resolve immediately to be able to think and feel beautifully. Biochemistry is very real and had a very obvious and profound effect within my system. That was undeniable.

The Motilium (Domperidone) that I took to stimulate my milk supply, worked pharmacologically by blocking dopamine which propelled me faster and further into my decline. Only through stopping the Motilium and trialling two medications, could I see my balance restore and I did achieve equilibrium again at that 11-week mark. As a disclaimer, this is not written to make you cease your medication if you are currently taking it for milk supply. This was merely my experience, and a conversation to be had with your prescribing physician about the best course of action for your individual situation.

I have recently listened to a podcast by Physio Laura, who had a lovely speaker Nikki McCahon who has created the *'dear mama project'* on Instagram. She had a four-part series about the journey to matrescence and I highly recommend it as a great listen! She explained that in a single pregnancy that a woman would have 1000 times the amount of oestrogen produced, compared to in one cycle and this equates to the ENTIRE amount of oestrogen produced in all of her cycles put together for the rest of her life! Wow!

Pregnancy produces 15 times the amount of progesterone than in one single cycle and brain image studies have shown that oxytocin, growth hormone, prolactin and relaxin can all *physically* change the brain structure.

When it is put in figuratively profound ways as this, it becomes undeniable and totally reasonable to understand the huge impact that this hormonal shift/cascade can have on someone with predispositions; and I also wonder about underlying biochemical/ nutritional predispositions.

Dr Oscar Serrallach's book *'The Postnatal Depletion Cure'* is another great read that discusses concepts surrounding underlying nutritional deficiencies, as well as neuro-inflammatory 'peptides' that cause disruption to the way our brain functions post birth and can cause certain symptoms.

I believe that if there are undeniable underlying deficiencies or imbalance during pre-pregnancy or pregnancy, that we can look at rectifying it through nutrition and targeted supplements. This perhaps may lessen the impact or allow it to last for a shorter period of time. Clinical trials and research are paramount in this moving forward, for our women in future generations.

My biochemical testing that I embarked upon after having Kaiyaan indicated a whole host of potential markers as possible predispositions for my post-natal depression, though not scientifically proven. I therefore cannot confidently ascertain full cause and effects at this stage but *very* passionate and interested in doing so. I was found to have:

- low levels of GABA (inhibitory neurotransmitter); which has been correlated with being produced by our gut microbiome, and low levels can be associated with anxiety
- low serotonin
- low tryptophan
- low morning cortisol
- low magnesium
- low zinc
- low iodine
- low selenium
- pyroluria (producing excess kryptopyrroles that bind to vitamin B6 and zinc to cause low levels of these; this is a hugely contentious topic in the medical field, so acknowledge this)
- MTFHR mutation (causing trouble with methylation of B-group vitamins)
- gluten intolerance/sensitivity
- high oxalates
- low B6
- oestrogen dominance
- two strains of high levels of bacteria in my gut that required treatment

My supplementation of these do require a good overhaul as they can make me nauseous, so I recommend working with a great Integrative GP and/or naturopath that has extensive experience and knowledge in this field. A lot of this testing is not subsidised by Medicare, so it can be a costly exercise that we want to make sure you are getting optimum outcomes from.

As to what specifically in these biochemical markers could have been rebalanced prior to pregnancy and what effect it would have on the outcome post-birth is so fascinating. Imagine the change in landscape moving forward in this whole area, if measurable and quantifiable markers could be shown and managed. I am truly so excited about this potentiality!

Another interesting point is the use of an epidural and whether that has any impact on adding to the biochemical cascade after birth. I did have an epidural with both of my boys and that was the only variable that was not different in each birth for me to know whether or not having one may have reduced my symptoms or delayed its onset?

Equally, I can appreciate that birth trauma is real with a painful and arduous natural birth. This can present its own host of healings necessary both physically, mentally and emotionally. Those women having caesareans have no choice but to have an epidural, so whilst this correlation may be interesting, I would not want any research to add any extra feelings of guilt for women that have PND and had an epidural. Yet, more an exercise of food for thought.

From a Western medicine perspective, it is very evident that taking my antidepressant increased my serotonin and noradrenaline, which brought me fully into my cognitive and full-capacity self. It took until 11 weeks post-partum for this effect to be seen, irrespective of me commencing a different medication at 6 to 7 weeks the first time, and commencing the one that did work much sooner at one week post-partum the second time. Once that imbalance was corrected, the fog was lifted and my body, mind and spirit felt as if they had returned and felt amazing!

From an Ayurvedic perspective, when we give birth our *Vata dosha* becomes aggravated, which is made of the elements of air and space. Specifically, the *Apana Vata* (which is a sub-set within the categorisation) undergoes extreme imbalance and aggravation. If this balance is not restored, nourished and nurtured, then our nervous systems become very aggravated and activate insomnia, anxiety, nervousness, depression, loss of appetite and a host of other symptoms.

Learning how to balance this aggravation through our diet, lifestyle, practices and mindfulness all form the foundation within Ayurveda to support the mother post-delivery. Strategies like eating warm, oily, heavier foods, spices to stimulate digestion and nourish the body, as well as practices to help keep the body moist/oily, warm, solid and grounded are some examples of what can be used.

Now we live in a society where the 'bouncing back to routine', and being out and about is worn as a badge of honour. Yet, Ayurveda encourages allowing space for nourishment and rest. We do not need to jump back into school drop offs and pickups, straight to our laptops writing out our next business plan and running the household as if having a baby was a routine dental check-up. Now is the time to call on our tribal and primal practices that are still deep within, and to lean on our community and tribe for the full support during this time in our life.

I would recommend that if you feel hormones may be a component to how you feel, then do seek the advice of an Integrative GP or GP, who can help you identify what areas can be balanced and help you to feel more aligned to health and well-being. They are a wealth of knowledge and through differential diagnosis, they can look after you holistically and advise the best course of action for you.

Certainly the appreciation and acknowledgement of the impact that hormones play on our biochemistry is the take home message here.

CHAPTER 6

MEDICATIONS

This topic is close to my heart for quite a number of reasons. The first being that because I am a pharmacist, I can completely appreciate their place in therapy and the science behind what they do in treating post-natal depression. Secondly, medications *absolutely* saved my life twice and I genuinely feel like I would not have made a strong recovery had I not commenced, committed and completed my course of treatment.

I want to dispel the myths and stigma that medications hold in treatment for post-natal depression, which I have seen first-hand during my practice in community pharmacy. Yet, also reading forums online and speaking with other mothers, it seems like people feel like it may be addictive, it may make them a zombie or numb their emotions. Whilst I do acknowledge that some women may feel this way, I would recommend being transparent with your physician to find the agent for you, as there is no one option fits all approach here.

My own experience was quite the contrary, where prior to medications having an effect, I was cold, distant, had no connection to emotion or had any feelings internally *at all*. I had switched off from the world at large and absolutely could not foster any cohesive thoughts or conversations with anybody, unless I spoke about my loop. Living with me would have been an absolute draining nightmare and I feel for my family for enduring it for as long as they all did.

Yet, once the medications had worked by increasing my serotonin and noradrenaline with some impact on dopamine with me stopping to take the Motilium for my milk supply (works by blocking dopamine); it was as if my light had returned. I immediately could think cohesively, the black fog that was all-consuming had disappeared and all of my capacity to feel had returned, *and* in abundance. It was such a profound effect that there is no way I could have gone on any longer in my previous state.

I was on the medication Lexapro for six months the first time and slowly weaned off thereafter, over the course of a month. I had no side effects whatsoever and I did not notice a thing whilst reducing dose. When I stopped completely, I still felt absolutely amazing.

The second time around I was on Pristiq, after trying the Lexapro first for almost 9 weeks. I was advised to stay on the Pristiq for twelve months, as it was considered a second relapse. It was recommended to remain on it longer to ensure that we did establish solid homeostasis within my system.

This is by no means a recommendation of what to or not to take. This is a conversation to be had with your prescribing physician and what will work for you is up to your symptoms, presentation and what your triage team feel is best suited for you; *if* they feel medication is what is needed, and is not always the case.

Whilst weaning off the Pristiq at the 12-month mark, I was advised by my doctor to do it slowly and to be kind and gentle to myself, as there were more noticeable physical side effects. She said to honour myself as if I were healing from surgery and to take it easy, and I truly appreciated her advice. I certainly experienced some 'brain zaps' which felt quite bizarre and would stop me in my tracks. This did take a good five to seven days until they subsided, but my mood did not change despite weaning, which was reassuring and a huge relief. It was helpful that my boys were older and not as demanding of me during that time, and I leant more on utilising creature comforts like takeaway and the T.V so I could just get through that time, which I did reasonably unscathed too, I might add.

Both times they had corrected my imbalance that the hormonal surges had brought on after birth. When I no longer needed them, my body was in perfect equilibrium so that their absence made no effect on my mood or how I was feeling.

The only thing that I noticed was that as a driver my confidence was so much more profound whilst on my medication than without. Perhaps the noradrenaline that it works to enhance, gave me more confidence and sense of ability compared to my baseline natural levels. I have especially noticed it in my driving since moving to Sydney where there are more people than I care to count, the drivers being more aggressive and spaces so incredibly tight!

Whilst I have picked up my pace, I do often wonder how my driving would be if I was still taking Pristiq, as sometimes after a particularly stressful drive I need to sit in my car and decompress for a few minutes. This most likely is due to my *Vata* aggravation as traffic, lots of movement and the hustle-bustle of a big city can induce this, so it may be a sign that I need to incorporate more *Vata* balancing activities to help nourish and soothe my nervous system. Or buy a Tesla that will drive itself...but then that will cause issues with my controlling aspect!

I can appreciate that finding the right medication that works can be exhausting, rather stressful and at times quite frustrating. Pharmacologically speaking it can take 1 to 3 weeks to see some improvement, 4 to 6 weeks to see a good effect and sometimes 6 to 8 weeks to see the *full* effects. During this 'waiting game', and it does feel that way for the patient and their family, everyone is waiting and hoping that this medication will provide some reprieve and respite, just like waiting to see if your ticket has won the lotto.

My first medication Valdoxan that I had taken for almost six weeks from around week 5 after having Ari, had no effect on my mood although, my sleep symptoms had improved, so it was not a complete waste of time. Yet, swapping over to my new medication Lexapro caused positive effect within 48 hours and only continued to improve over the next few weeks.

The second time, I went straight onto Lexapro thinking that it would exert the same effect again. I was on it for around nine weeks including a doubling of the dosage during this time and adding additional agents, but then my team decided to make a change after this amount of time elapsing. After this swapping of medication again, within a matter of a few days of commencing after weaning the first, the second one worked and for both PND's I had returned 'back to life' as I call it at the 11 week mark.

This 'waiting game' certainly can be an anxious time in not knowing if or when it will work. Also waiting the full six to eight weeks with no improvement can add strain and pressure onto the patient, but also the relationships within the home. As a society we are very solution oriented and very much into 'quick fixes' with looking for very definite cause and effect solutions. I am that person. Yet, in the nature of the beast that is, this is a game of patience and perseverance and also of establishing faith in something greater than oneself, as a means to keep on going.

It was through my experience of this arduous 'waiting game', that aside from wanting to remove the fear to seek help and to break through the stigma of starting medications, I also wanted to provide support tools to heal the *Vata* imbalance that was occurring *whilst* waiting for Western treatments to work. Using tools and practices that balance this aggravation within the system, as well as redirecting energy into high vibration and mindful practices to exert subtle healing, my hope is that the waiting is not so painful and torturous. I literally would sit in my room like a hermit or leper waiting for the magic miracle to occur and shift, all the while feeling so lonely and trapped in this dark reality.

I also can understand the concerns and fears with different medications and their safety with breastfeeding. The one good thing about my breastfeeding journey was that medication choice was not a factor for my treatment plan and I did not have that extra factor to consider. Yet, I can completely appreciate the hesitation and concern for breastfeeding women. Thankfully as a pharmacist we are privy to up-to-date information all around the safety of medications, herbs and alcohol when breastfeeding. Discussing this concern with your physician or pharmacist, can allow them to make the choice of treatment most suitable for you.

My hope and intention is that my Wholeistic Healing Co. website can provide mothers with a search tool to ascertain the safety profile of medication, over-the-counter medications and herbs with breastfeeding and also the safety of combining alcohol with medication, so that people can make informed decisions with their health and safety always at the forefront.

I know that with conscious living and a lot of people wanting to live in a manner that is 'low-tox', medication may seem to go against this lifestyle choice. My point that I will strongly advocate for is, that post-natal depression can be a life or death situation, and medications unequivocally saved my life. There is no point to living in a low-tox manner, if you are not living to experience it. I believe there is a time and place for everything and I strongly believe that safety concerns over starting medications need to be debunked from the inside out.

We cannot live in a world that is so black or white, where we choose only Eastern *or* only Western modalities. The synergy and optimum outcome and harmony is through the best application of both. We need to understand that not all science is 'bad' and not all holistic practices are 'good' or proven, and vice versa. We need to move forward not living in such extreme ends and to find the cohesive balance between the two.

I touched on the fact that a lot of people may perceive that their personalities can change, they become 'numb' or that the medications are addictive or habit-forming. For me, it allowed me to return to my normal state of functioning and out of the numb and zombie version in my PND. I fully agree that it is important to be observant with how you are feeling within yourself when commencing medication. Through the contrast between the darkness and feeling your light within, you will know how it is working.

It is also very important to seek feedback as to how you are responding, functioning and behaving from your spouse or partner. You may not be able to feel or see tangible changes, or what you perceive to be a different personality, because you have been in a depressive state for so long that you may have lost sense of what you were like before. Use the sounding board and visuals from your family around you, to let you know how you have been since starting medication. Allow them to acknowledge how you are progressing as a way of assessing how well treatment is working, in addition to how you feel within yourself.

Another important issue is the concern or fear that being on anti-depressants, being diagnosed and hence 'labelled' as having post-natal depression will permanently be on one's health record. The fear that it will affect how employers view you or your insurances, is one that I have heard before. Specifically, for health professionals I have several colleagues across multiple branches of medicine and have had multiple conversations about the state of mental health and the fear associated with speaking out about it. There is a resounding fear that being 'labelled' in a certain way will impact their registration and how 'fit' they are perceived in practising.

If the fear of losing our children or positions were not at risk, then perhaps speaking out about mental illness would prevail. If we, as a society, do not just *say* that it is OK to speak out but actually *allow* for all aspects to be clear and free to reach out and access support, then perhaps others will feel supported and held in a beautiful way. I say this categorically for mothers but also for health professionals that I see a common thread in as well.

It is by replacing the fear with more understanding and empathy. This awareness, especially in a world of Covid, where figures of depression and anxiety have and will continue to rise with the continuing stress and strain on our way of life, is of utmost importance. I stand up for mothers and health professionals alike to say that it is OK to not be OK, and to stand up for more support and reform.

HEALTH TIP:

ACRONYM FOR SURVIVING THIS PERIOD

<u>A</u>	_Ask for help from your partner, family and friends_
<u>R</u>	_Reach out for help from health professionals_
<u>M</u>	_Make a commitment statement to yourself and keep it with you to keep accountability_
<u>E</u>	_Exercise; make it a daily priority not for weight loss or exertion but for your endorphins and well-being_
<u>R</u>	_Rest when your body tells you to and partake in rejuvenation practices to heal your body_

WHAT ARE SOME PRACTICAL TIPS TO GET THROUGH THIS PERIOD?

+ Sign up to a meal train with other mothers or people in your community

+ Sign up to a meal delivery service who delivers freshly made food with prana (life-force) rich produce

+ Do online groceries delivered to your home (ideally not during nap time)

+ Bulk order items you know that you will always need and use; pantry staples, nappies, wipes etc.

+ Hire a cleaner if finances allow for it; they can change bedding, fold washing, clean etc.

+ Prepare snacks for the week if possible to make sure you never get hungry

+ Delegate tasks to your partner or family if they live locally. Do not be shy or embarrassed to ask for help...now is the time!

+ See if friends can arrange play dates for your older child so you can rest and they don't get bored

+ Sleep whenever you can. Turn off the T.V, phone, doorbell and just sleep. Your body will thank you

+ Write down niggles/concerns and find solutions with your partner so they don't continue to annoy you

+ Drink lots of water, especially if you are breastfeeding. Dehydration can give you a headache and make you feel cloudier than you already do. Avoid cold/icy water and stick with ideally warm water as this will best support your digestive fire from an Ayurvedic perspective

+ Do your pelvic floor exercises as often as you can; perhaps every feed and nappy time. Literally 'squeeze' it in as much as you can throughout your day. Get a women's health physiotherapist to assess your pelvic floor health after the 6-week mark to get specific guidance into what exercises will best support your recovery

HEALTH TIP:

*WHAT ARE PREDISPOSING FACTORS FOR
GETTING POSTNATAL DEPRESSION?*

*Although there is no concrete definitive cause of post-natal depression, the
following are a list of predisposing factors listed from the PANDA (Perinatal
Anxiety and Depression Australia) website;*

+ Family or personal history of anxiety or depression

+ Traumatic birth

+ Birth disappointment

+ Relationship difficulties

+ Controlling or abusive behaviour

+ Family violence

+ Stressful life events

+ A troubled pregnancy

+ Fertility issues or previous pregnancy loss

+ Past history of abuse

+ Lack of social support

+ Financial difficulties

CHAPTER 7

SELF-HELP STRATEGIES
FOR THE MOTHER

For those of you who are currently in the thick of it and in the depths of darkness, firstly beautiful Mamma I see you, I feel what you are going through and feel *so* proud of you for reaching out for help! I promise you that there IS light at the end of the tunnel and you just need to have faith in yourself and know that you are powerful beyond measure and you _will_ get through this chapter. I promise.

Each day for me was long, anxiety ridden and filled with talking about my loop to whoever would listen. If they didn't listen, then I would spend my days sitting in an empty room in absolute silence. I could sit in there all day in the guise of trying to sleep but would just ruminate through my anxiety ridden thoughts. Each hour felt like an eternity and each day I just wanted to hide under the blankets and disappear from this reality *completely*.

I felt lonely.

I felt scared.

I felt hopeless.

I genuinely thought there was nothing that could make any of this better and that I would be stuck in this reality forever. This was even after knowing that I had recovered from the first post-natal depression. Yet, my body was completely taken over by this horrible dis-ease that I truly did not feel like there was a way out. I felt like I was drowning and could not breathe.

The pain was *palpable*.

The anxiety pain was painful too.

I felt *completely* trapped.

I did however, hold on for my boys and the primal feeling that I had to hold on and heal myself for *them*. I could not leave my husband with two boys even though my ideations were rampant and I felt like running away and never coming back. Yet, my heart *always* stayed beating for my boys and I knew that it would be the cruelest thing to do, to not heal and leave all of this behind. I had to dig deep for *every tiny* ounce of courage and strength to keep my head out of the quicksand and breathe life into my days moment by moment. Looking back, it truly was such a horrible and painful time.

The love for my boys kept me going and *they* were the *reason why* I held on each and every day.

I ask that you write a <u>commitment statement</u> and write your 'why' that you can look at whenever you need a reminder. You could give it to your partner so that they can help keep you on track and accountable for taking steps forward in your healing journey. Read the statement back to yourself as often as you need, to remind yourself of *where* you would like to be and *what* you are willing to do in order to reach that point. It will remind you of all your reasons for holding on and it will get you through each long and relenting day, when you fall or feel like it is all too hard. I felt like that daily.

Sometimes every hour. Yet, I picked myself up every time and though I felt hopeless, I knew that I had people who needed me.

I find that physical conditions can have very quantifiable strategies or milestones to track your progress. Surgery usually has a beautiful aspect to it where your body innately heals, so the next day by natural law (granted there are no complications) will be better and then better again after that. I have had an umbilical hernia repaired as well as surgery on my toes since having Kaiyaan. I would say that surgeons giving a crystal clear outline of what to expect at each week and advising when I could do what, *helped* in an amazing way. I was able to gauge my progress in a very logical and quantifiable way. I knew what to expect.

However, with psychology and healing of this nature there is no black and white prescription, nor a clear-cut masculine timeline as to exactly *what* will make you better and *when* you will start to *feel* better. The not knowing when I would recover was the hardest part for all of us, and we had to hold onto faith to keep us going. Even when there were times we had lost faith completely, we had to dig deep and keep going.

I have created/listed tools below specifically for what I wished I had done during my recovery, *instead* of sitting in my closed room *waiting* for some magical thing to happen to me. I was waiting for western treatments to work but made the 11 weeks truly painful for myself and everyone involved. I felt like I could not take the reins in finding what I needed to do, nor could I take the initiative into actioning it.

Using any or all of these strategies could have a cumulative effect to bring about inner nourishment and rejuvenation within your body and to calm your aggravated nervous system. It most certainly would have filled my days with action steps and allow for subtle respite within my body. It also would have been a *far* more pleasant experience within the home for all of us, instead of me sitting alone festering on my incessant thoughts. I hope that the list below will give you some guidance into finding some respite and lightness for you, your family and in your home.

Utilise any or all that resonate within you, on any or all of the days.

For any partners or family members reading this on behalf of your loved one, use these strategies in your home and literally *be* the initiative to allow these steps to be actioned. I was given the space and time to heal, yes, but I wished someone had taken the reins for me and literally set things up and almost forced me to do things, other than sit in my room. I could not make decisions nor take action steps myself, so I needed someone to spell out what to do and help me do it, which is what I hope this can achieve for your beautiful women.

I would also say that a lot of these points or strategies can be utilised if you are suffering from anxiety and depression during your pregnancy as well as post-natal depression; so the entire PNDA period. Obviously points about alcohol consumption should be zero, and watching the caffeine consumption also during pregnancy. However, on the whole, a lot of these strategies both from a Western and Eastern paradigm are relevant and can be so helpful in managing your symptoms and how you feel.

SUMMARY LIST OF ACTION STEPS

1. CBT, IPT, MBCT or Behavioural therapy at a GP or psychologist. Seek medical treatment
2. Manage self-talk and thoughts
3. Working through problem solving
4. Exercise (all exercise, yoga and Ayurvedic yoga)
5. Reduce alcohol to minimal level, if not completely
6. Stay hydrated and reduce caffeine

7. Manage stress (meditation, breathing/Pranayama, a warm bath, grounding activities and scents, access your unique relaxation tool kit of strategies)
8. Reach out to a friend or family member to talk
9. Do something that you normally love to do that sparks you up
10. Turn off the T.V and unnecessary noise or stimulation
11. Support yourself with as much sleep as possible
12. Ayurvedic food, Ayurvedic teas and herbs/spices (Prana – life-force rich food, little to no processed and convenience type foods)
13. Ayurvedic practices (massage, things taken in through the 5 senses)
14. Infant massage as a bonding and connective activity
15. Create an environment conducive to healing
16. Stop worrying about others
17. Be gentle on yourself
18. Gratitude
19. Go out in nature, break up the routine

WHAT ARE THE SELF-HELP STRATEGIES FOR THE MOTHER?

1. SEEK MEDICAL HELP: CBT, IPT, MBCT OR BEHAVIOURAL THERAPY WITH A GP OR PSYCHOLOGIST

The first and *most* important step to take, is to acknowledge that you are not feeling yourself after having a baby and to make an appointment to see your doctor. This is most likely the hardest step, but the *most important* to getting you onto your road of recovery. Waiting for it to get better on its own or being in denial that you are feeling fine, is what will keep you in this situation for longer.

Speak with your obstetrician or GP and ask for a long or double appointment, in order to get a Mental Health Plan drawn up and a referral made to a psychologist and/or psychiatrist. I would say to ask for perinatal specific specialists, as this is their niche area of practice. Though if they are fully booked, then gain access to whoever is first available to expedite the process. They will welcome you into their room with an open heart and will take the reins of finding you the most suitable care, in order for you to make a strong recovery from this. This can help you speak openly without judgement as to how you are feeling and how to best navigate a treatment plan for your recovery.

Do not hold back on anything you are feeling so that they can refer you to *exactly* who you need to see. Be honest. Take your partner or a family member if this would help. Otherwise leave the baby with someone whilst you chat without any interruption with your doctor. I would also say to write down a list of questions and points that you want to discuss with the doctor before going. This will make you feel less anxious and stressed about the appointment, as well as allow you to get the most out of the appointment and gain access to the best of help that you require.

Upon getting an appointment to see a psychologist and/or psychiatrist, they can review your situation and what course of treatment will be most suited to you. They can help talk through any birth trauma, PTSD, feelings, emotions, mindsets and self-talk patterns, as well as provide amazing coping strategies to help you in whatever way you need.

They may offer CBT (Cognitive Behavioural Therapy), IPT (Interpersonal Therapy) or MBCT (Mindfulness-Based Cognitive Therapy) as ways to unveil all that they need to, and give you amazing strategies to work through areas of concern for you. They also have a whole range of treatments, tools and strategies including medication and ECT (Electroconvulsive Therapy). Trust in your physician in choosing the best options for you, as they will piece together your presenting symptoms, past medical history, and construct the *best* treatment protocol specific to you.

Release any feelings you may have about starting medication if this is something they recommend, as well as any hang-ups you may have about starting therapy. You should only be given praise for reaching out and saying that you know you are not feeling well and want to get better. You wouldn't think twice to see a physiotherapist if you sprained your ankle, and this is NO different. Go in with an open mind and open heart.

Another important point if you are having repetitive thoughts, is to try your absolute best to find an outlet other than speaking about it, unless it is to your health professional. Ask your doctor for *specific strategies* for your unique circumstance to help with how you can *best* manage your symptoms and loop, whilst you are waiting for treatments to take effect. Talking about it only seeks to reinforce the thoughts and strengthening the depression that you are in. I know I felt as if I could explode when no one listened to me, when all I wanted to do was talk about it. Yet, my doctor had given strict instructions to cut it off, so that it would allow me a chance to redirect my thoughts and come out of this perpetual cycle.

Distract yourself or dedicate a time once a day to get it off your chest, then go back to your commitment statement that you wrote and somehow pull yourself away from the ruminating thoughts. This is where friends and family can be saviours at redirecting your energy and where it is being channelled. Go for a walk in that moment or listen to some music. Just shift that thought away from the loop.

Another point with Western treatment, is the awareness that it may take time to start working and it may not be a 'quick-fix'. However, knowing this will allow you to be patient as well as utilise other strategies to help calm your aggravated nervous system, *whilst* you are waiting for these treatments to work. My hope is that this 'waiting game' becomes less painful, utilising the strategies below. However, I encourage you to access Western treatment modalities as soon as possible, so that your balance can be corrected sooner rather than later.

Rest assured that taking this first step may be the hardest but upon doing so, you are walking closer to finding the best solution for you. Be patient, hold faith and stay committed in your recovery and the rest *will* unfold perfectly.

2. MANAGE SELF-TALK AND THOUGHTS
Though easier said than done, if you start to observe your thoughts and mindfully change the direction of them, you can create new neural pathways in thoughts that support you. You want them to serve you instead of bring you down. Speak with your healthcare team for *specific* strategies for your situation and their guidance will help you navigate through this self-talk path. This may allow more positive thoughts to infiltrate your system and alter the way in which you respond and perceive certain situations.

When you observe yourself, jot the observation down in case you forget it. Then if it pops up again, you will most likely spot it more easily and identify certain patterns or triggers in your thinking. Swapping a negative spin to a positive spin eventually changes the lens through which we view life. Spot yourself thinking 'why do I find this so hard? Everyone else finds it so easy, I must be a terrible Mum' and stop. Take a deep breath and rephrase it 'I am finding it hard, but many other Mums feel this way too. I should ask someone'. This observation and changing the trajectory of the thought is very powerful and can alter the way in which you respond in the world as you move on, not just through this chapter.

On a more spiritual perspective and not to confuse you any more than you may already be with all that is going on! Yet, I ask that if you are observing certain thoughts when they pop up, then ask yourself who is the observer and who is the real you? The real you, your *true* self is the one 'observing' your thoughts and your thoughts/mind are not in fact you at all, though it does feel that way now.

Trust me, I've been there! This little perspective may allow you to realise that thoughts are just thoughts, and the true self within you lies beneath those thoughts. They are *just* thoughts and thoughts can be changed! Allow that to help focus your healing and attention to nurture and nourish this true self within, and do not get fixated or taken for a rollercoaster ride with your thoughts. Sell your tickets and hop on the ride within.

3. WORKING THROUGH PROBLEM SOLVING

This exercise can be done alone to help filter and clear your thoughts, or you may prefer to work through this with your partner or another family member. Every thought that is troubling you, and you are placing a lot of time and energy towards, write it down and then brainstorm possible solutions for them. This allows the energy to be directed towards the solving and resolving of the issues, rather than watering the problem and hoping that it will not grow.

More often than not, venting the problem and working out solutions can be a very productive exercise. You may feel lighter with the problem shared or out of your system. Often hearing another person's perspective may shine the light in a way you could not have even predicted.

Another cathartic process may be once you have written your thoughts down, then shred the paper into little pieces. That way, it is no longer relevant or deserving of your energy, now that solutions have been worked through.

The above may work for most problems and yet, serious and heavy problems such as a sick child or parent may not be as easy to find an actual solution. The very act of bringing your feelings and concerns to the forefront, allows your feelings to be heard and validated. Your partner may simply hold you and this may allow you to feel completely safe and nurtured. Whilst no magical solution has been found, the very act of being held has allowed you to feel the support that you need. Don't be shy or embarrassed to ask for the space and time to do this, as you deserve to feel lighter from such an activity.

Journaling is another way to articulate your thoughts and feelings and it can be a very effective way of being an outlet for any recurring or residual feelings within. Getting a beautiful journal book that you can spend time in writing in a safe and energetically clear space, can help to heal any feelings you may not even realise are lying buried within.

I have used a journal since I was a little girl of 6 or 7 years old. It first started in a 'Dear God' prayer manner and slowly progressed in different styles of what worked for me in various phases of my life. I have written in very deep articulate forms, as well as writing questions, then writing whatever was in my heart and mind pertaining to getting to the root cause.

Since having my boys, I may not get a chance to write in my journal even weekly, or it may be a quick scramble of thoughts just to realign my thought process, act as a boxing bag, a quick outlet or just dot points to literally purge any quick or pertinent thoughts that I have. Yet, it is always on my night stand or dining table so I know exactly where my tool is when I need it and I have access to utilising it whenever I feel compelled or called to it.

I find it very therapeutic and I often get intuitive guidance in solutions or finding the underlying reason for certain feelings, so it has been a very powerful healing tool for me. I have always thought of myself as an introvert for this inner reflection activity; though I get fuelled and re-energised through connection and conversations with others, so I feel like I may be a harmonious mix of both. I need my solitude, quiet time and space but I need that social connection to release my inner energy...try it and see if you find it helpful too.

4. EXERCISE

I feel like exercise is highly underrated and through its ability to enhance endorphins, serotonin, circulation and oxygenation through the body, in as little as even 20 minutes, it will undoubtedly make you feel better than before you did a workout!

Of course after having a baby, I would not advise you to go for a run or start training for a marathon. However, if your doctor has given you the all clear to go walking, then I would start there. Pelvic floor health would be most crucial as the risk of prolapse or implications from downward exerting is pertinent during the early stages, as well as the physical recovery from childbirth and a C-section healing. Therefore, do ask your OB first and I would highly recommend the use of a women's health physiotherapist to help guide you towards the safest time and means of starting your exercise journey.

However, going for beautiful walks as a starting point has so many benefits. The fresh air, seeing other people around and connecting yourself into the world around you again can be so powerful, especially if you have been locked away in a hospital, your bedroom or house since delivering. There is something *so* healing about being in nature and feeling the fresh air on your skin and through your lungs. Take your pram and partner too, so you can all benefit from the magical effects of exercise!

From an Ayurvedic perspective with our *Vata* imbalance after birth and keeping in mind that *Vata* is made up of air and space, then we want to make some modifications. Especially if it is during Autumn and Winter, then we need to be more mindful in making these modifications.

Try to keep your body warm, especially your head and ears by wearing a beanie so too much air and wind cannot enter your ears. If you can wear a scarf and keep your body warm, that is most beneficial. Make sure your feet are warm with socks and that you are wearing protective and warming shoes and not open thongs. Walk at a comfortable pace and one that is not going to make you exhausted or be too vigorous, but enough to feel the oxygenation and blood pumping freely in your body.

Add to your exercise as your body feels it can comfortably manage. Do what feels uplifting but not exhausting you further. The aim is not a crash weight loss and drill sergeant regime, but rather enough to uplift your feel-good hormones and make a positive shift in your internal biochemistry.

YOGA

Utilising Ayurvedic Yoga which has sequences to support an aggravated *Vata dosha* will be a beautiful practice to allow movement, flexibility, build strength as well as calming the mind through focus. *Pranayama* (breathing), *asana* (yoga poses) and the integration component of *Savasana* (typically known as the 'relaxation' portion at the end of the class, which helps to integrate the learnings from the practice), all help to strengthen and centre both body and mind.

My studies of Ayurvedic Yoga have allowed me to appreciate the modifications of asana to best support heating the body, grounding and calming the nervous system. Mindfully choosing sequences, holding lengths, the way we modify the *asana* specific for the *Vata dosha* is very therapeutic in restoring balance within the body. We can also utilise specific *Pranayama* (breathing) for maximum therapeutic effect within the body.

233

I aim to utilise my training to create Yoga teachings specifically for *Vata* imbalance and to make these suitable for pregnancy and for all women post-birth to help support their bodies and minds in the most specifically-tailored way. I find this modality so connective and therapeutic in bringing about harmony within our system. I am so grateful to be learning this content and so excited to bring it to the world as a necessary healing modality for all women!

Other beautiful areas that Ayurvedic Yoga utilise are the use of mantra and colours to best support the *Vata dosha*. The mantras of RAM, SHRIM, OM and HRIM can produce a specific effect within the body through its vibration and holding focus on it for the scattered *Vata* mind.

The use of colours to help support the *Vata dosha* through wearing clothes or having imagery in art works or with flowers around you, can help to exert balancing of an aggravated *dosha* after childbirth.

Colours that are supportive to a *Vata dosha* include utilising warm, earthy tones;

    i.   Warm and sunny yellow, orange and red
    ii.   Browns
    iii.   Deep red, deep orange and gold
    iv.   Warm pastels
    v.   Sunny greens

Colours that are best avoided to support the *Vata dosha* include dark colours such as black and cooling colours such as blue.

I love that simple, mindful choices utilising all of our senses in Ayurveda exert subtle therapeutic balancing within our body. Subtle effects all add up to creating a sense of well-being within the body, which can be beneficial whilst waiting for Western allopathic treatments to start working. They can also be utilised throughout your life moving forward knowing that it will support your system to feeling the best that it can, especially if living in a city or you have a busy lifestyle with lots of movement. Moving to Sydney I find myself having to utilise *Vata* balancing practices to reduce the effects of our fast-pace city and way of life here. Though Sydney is home, it requires my body to recalibrate to its fast intensity and I can feel the effects of the fast movement within my system and adjust my practices accordingly. A very empowering tool.

Other traditional yoga that would support a woman with *Vata* imbalance after birth include the practices of;

+ Slow Vinyasa
+ Yin Yoga
+ Restorative Yoga
+ Satyananda Yoga
+ Kundalini Yoga

As long as you feel able physically, get the all-clear from your physician; start slowly and work your way up based on your level. Exercise in any form is so beneficial to our body, mind and spirit. I utilise it throughout my day to help give energy bursts and relieve stress; especially more so during Covid lockdowns with my boys and fur-baby. Wearing active wear means that you are ready at any moment to be active and exercise without using extra thought processes as to when you can do it. You are rearing to go 24/7, which takes out aspects of the motivation factor! Well that's my excuse for always being in active wear anyway!

If I feel like I have entered into a funk, which does happen based on my diet, lifestyle practices, how much I am working, our business stress...and how grating I find Sydney traffic, then I use exercise as the tool to help lift me out of my funk. It works very successfully and I always feel better after working out; whether it is a walk, run, strength training at home or going to the gym. Let's just say that I have never felt worse after a workout compared to before walking into it!

I have purchased Kayla Itsines' BBG program, Sarah Boulazeris's Bumpfit program and Sharny and Julius' programs also throughout my years. I also follow Emily Skye and Rachel Finch as I enjoy their content too. We are so lucky that there are so many exciting exercise programs to utilise in the comfort of our own home, and I have thoroughly enjoyed partaking in them and being part of their community.

Find what you resonate with and carve out the time you deserve to feel amazing! I aim to move my body for 30 minutes as a minimum every day. Immediately I feel more clarity in my mind, more agile and energy levels go sky high. The days that I skip out on it, I can feel the difference with how I feel so try my absolute best to move!

When I recovered from both of my surgeries after having Kaiyaan, I found the 6 weeks of not being able to exercise very challenging. It took about 3 months after both to restore to 'full-capacity', which I revelled in, being able to move my body again at that point. Similar to mental health, when physical abilities are compromised it becomes so much easier to feel the gratitude of full health and function being restored to all its glory. Our bodies are our vehicle in life, let us fuel them with nourishing food and beautiful movement to get the most out of life...plus the effect on biochemistry is undeniably necessary in this PND period!

5.   REDUCE ALCOHOL TO MINIMAL LEVEL, IF NOT COMPLETELY
After a long pregnancy it may feel like a dream to drink alcohol to help celebrate or calm your anxiety, especially if that is a predominate symptom. However, alcohol in itself acts as a depressant and may work to compound your feelings of depression and darkness. By having a cumulative effect of depressants, it can hinder your progress.

My Dad has always had a saying that 'what is like nectar in the beginning is like poison in the end' and vice versa. In this instance, alcohol may seem like a beautiful treat or luxury (i.e. the nectar) but it may end up keeping you held in depression for longer than you would like (i.e. the poison).

Also there is the possibility of alcohol potentiating or affecting any prescription medication that you have been given for your PND. Alcohol can enhance drowsiness, dizziness and the effects of your medication. Sometimes it can produce fatal outcomes such as respiratory depression, so vigilant care and attention are required here and I would always discuss alcohol with your prescribing physician, to get specific guidance on your exact circumstances and treatment.

My Dad's saying of 'what is like poison in the beginning is like nectar in the end' works here, where it may seem like not drinking is so difficult and restrictive coming out of a 9-month hiatus. Yet, abstaining for a little while longer may allow your medications to work fully and to allow for healing to occur even more effectively.

Whilst I enjoy having a few drinks with friends and on the weekend, I am mindfully aware that I function so much better with less in my body. However, when I drink I enjoy the process and do not add any extra emotional *Ama* or toxins, by feeling guilty when drinking. I enjoy it with the joy and fun that it is shared with friends and I do not beat myself up about having it.

When you are well enough again to add alcohol into your system, take care if you are still taking medication; whether it be over-the-counter or prescription. Enjoy it as a treat within limits and let go of any hang ups about it, so that it is only an experience shared with joy and friendships and it is a beautiful celebration of life.

Make sure you stay within the NHMRC recommended alcohol guidelines, which currently stand at women having no more than 10 standard drinks a week and no more than four standard drinks on any one day, after you have made your recovery. Breastfeeding would require further considerations to be made with respect to timings with feeding.

6. STAY HYDRATED AND REDUCE CAFFEINE

Our bodies are made up of 70 percent water in certain areas and we are designed to maintain optimum hydration, so that all of our bodily systems can function well. If we are dehydrated we can compound our feelings of a foggy head, dizziness and feeling lethargic. Depression also has symptoms like these, so if we are not looking after our basic human needs of hydration, more if you are breastfeeding or exercising, then we can enhance these symptoms. Though seemingly simple, it is an important part of healing after having a baby to flush out all of the toxins and to support our adrenergic, renal and liver systems as our detox organs.

From an Ayurvedic perspective, the recommendation is to drink hot if not warm water, rather than cold or cool water. Cold water can extinguish our digestive fire and drinking too close to meal times can impair or reduce our ability to best digest and assimilate our food. We want to best support our digestion, as it is an important aspect around our wellbeing and ability to prevent disease.

Caffeine is a stimulant so consuming this in excess if you are having symptoms of anxiety, restlessness and insomnia can make it worse or exacerbate your symptoms. Caffeine can be found in tea, green tea, coffee and chocolate. Similar to alcohol, if you have been restricting how much caffeine you drink during your pregnancy, then it may feel like a beautiful luxury that you have been counting down to drink at your pre-pregnancy levels.

I would say to start slowly and monitor how you are feeling when starting caffeine. If you are finding that it is elevating your heart rate, affecting your sleep, or making you feel anxious or irritable, then certainly reduce its consumption and replace it with decaf or herbal options. It is also very dehydrating so will mean that your water consumption will need to compensate for this effect.

Be mindful of the timing that you consume caffeine, as for some people anything after midday can affect sleep and others can be fine to have it much later in the day. Research has suggested that 2pm is the 'cut-off' time. Observation is your friend here. It is a good habit to have when breastfeeding, as a way to see how what you are eating and drinking is affecting your baby. As a pharmacist that would often be my strategy in trying to ascertain what allergies or reactions a baby would have, based on what the mother would eat; so this can be applied in this situation as well.

7. MANAGE STRESS
Stress with a newborn is inevitable even to the most monk-like person! I dare anyone who feels like they can handle a tremendous amount of stress to stay with a newborn and time how long it cracks even the most serene person. We are human and I can appreciate the idealism in this strategy, as we all aspire to respond more calmly to stimuli or situations, and it may not be the easiest of feats to overcome!

Coupled with already having feelings of anxiety and depression from our altered biochemistry, an aggravated nervous system due to our *Vata* aggravation and imbalance post-birth, stress can certainly be a factor that can hinder our healing by stretching an already stretched nervous system…and that sounds like an awful lot of stretching!

There will be some stressors that unfortunately fall out of our control. Covid would be a perfect example of this. Other examples could be your partner losing their job, financial stress or an illness or death within the family. Life does not stop because we have children nor because we have post-natal depression; but this is where adopting strategies to help us cope better with stress is wonderful, as well as leaning on lifelines of support in any ways you can receive it.

Yet, it is important to understand that our nervous systems *are* stretched after having a baby and there is more tendency to have hyper-sensitive reactions to noise, stimuli and stressors. It becomes so much more critical or crucial to fully embrace mindfulness techniques, calmness strategies and practices that assist you to feel more grounded and centred. Here are a few listed below:

MEDITATION

Meditation is an amazing strategy that allows our attention to be focused on breath, a mantra or single pointed imagery and it can produce a vast array of changes in our minds. Jay Shetty, has his own podcast and his book *'Think Like a Monk'* where he discusses the importance and benefits of meditation and what impact it does make on our minds and the brain makeup itself. I love all of his podcasts so I would highly recommend him for support tools.

Dr Joe Dispenza is another resource who I have leaned on and teaches all about the ability to rewire our mind and neural pathways, through meditation and mindfulness techniques. He has several books and meditations that are available and I would recommend looking at his work if your mind and hearts allow for it.

Guided meditations I personally have found effective for myself as my very active, running *Vata/Pitta* mind is always moving and jumping to the next thought and the next thought. By following the words and imagery of a guided meditation, it has allowed me to focus my attention more effectively and I have gained a lot from it.

I have created a number of guided meditations and healing tracks through my Wholeistic Healing Co. website working with Listening to Smile, each having a very specific focus. All have certain healing frequencies, binaural beats and tones to promote relaxation and specific functions based on the intention. I have meditations to listen to when you are feeding your baby with the intention of love and nourishment, as well as for helping with sleep, together with subconscious connection affirmations, gratitude tracks, releasing anger/guilt/shame and fear as well as relaxation of the nervous system.

Take some time out for yourself in a quiet and calm environment and make the space how you like it to be. Meditate however you choose to, for as little as 5 minutes if that time is what you are able to dedicate. Work your way up if you can and allow it to nourish your nervous system and bring calm into your being.

Smiling Mind and Insight Timer are others examples of great tools for meditations which I encourage you to work through if it resonates with you. Mindfulness whilst quite a trending word, has been encouraged for eons. In the modern world that we live in, it has become a necessity to soothe our nervous system to ensure that it does not short circuit and spiral us into feeling overwhelmed. Do not feel discouraged into thinking there is a 'right' or 'wrong' way to do it.

Make some space in your home and time to allow yourself to partake in mindfulness, in whatever way feels authentic to you. In time, you will find your groove and what best resonates with you to feel calm and centred. For me, I love to light a candle, play my healing frequency music and either focus on my breath or do a guided meditation. I do it at night once the boys are asleep or listen to an audio with earphones as I lie in bed. Each day looks a little different but making time for myself to do it, always makes me feel more centred and aligned in doing so.

BREATHING/ PRANAYAMA

Deep and slow breathing can reduce our stress and anxiety by expanding our diaphragm and chests. This activates our parasympathetic nervous system instead of our active and stimulated sympathetic nervous system, which is our survival system.

It is a very effective mindfulness technique and can bring about calm in any situation and environment you are in, no matter where you are or what time of the day! It is silent (mostly) too which is most helpful with a sleeping baby that you do not want to wake!

Pranayama is one of the Eight Limbs of Yoga and is the practice of clearing energy channels within the body through breath. There are several different types that you can do as a way to connect your body, mind and spirit. Though you do not need to be a yogi to practise mindful and therapeutic *Pranayama*, I mention this because there must be some truth to the relaxation and mindfulness that it brings, if yogis and monks utilise this strategy alike.

I would recommend that several times throughout the day, where just like your thoughts and tone in which you speak with yourself, be the observer of your breath and notice whether it is deep, considered and diaphragmatic. Or it is fast, shallow and centred around the chest? Both of these have very different feelings associated with them. We want to utilise big, slow, mindful, deep, diaphragmatic breaths as a way to calm our nervous systems and activate our relaxation response.

In times of stress, I always find that my breath is shallow and based in my chest area rather than being deliberate and deep in nature, so I can tell how I am feeling just by noticing how I am breathing in that moment.

Try doing these observations at set times throughout the day or you could do it when you notice you are feeling overwhelmed and starting to respond to the stress around you. It is also a practice of connection as it allows your mind to be the observer of what your body is doing and you become aware that who you truly are is the person observing all of this. THAT is empowering!

A *Pranayama* called *Nadi Shodhana*, which is alternate nostril breathing is an excellent calming tool. By alternating deep breaths in through one nostril and out of the other, by using your thumb and ring finger to hold the right and left nostril closed respectively if using your right hand, with your index and middle finger on your third eye; it works to calm a *Vata* aggravated system. It is very relaxing and quite invigorating also, as you feel the oxygenation in the brain which feels amazing! I personally love doing this in the morning.

There are a host of other *Pranayama's* that all exert a specific effect within the body. I would not stress about learning all of them in the depths of your depression but if you have practised some, or if you focus on very deliberate and mindful breathing, then it will convey some therapeutic effects in your body and bring about relaxation and support your nervous system in feeling more calm. If you do have access and are able to learn more about it, then it will be a very helpful tool to use.

With breathing, I have put some detailed information about what to do if you are experiencing a panic attack within Chapter 1 of Part 2. Breathing is a wonderful foundation for being able to work through anxiety and a panic attack, so I encourage you to look through there again for some other helpful strategies utilising breath work.

243

A WARM BATH

This can be very healing and nourishing to our bodies as it will feel held by the water, hydrated and completely filled with lightness. Whilst these tips may appear simple, if someone can take the reins and encourage you to immerse yourself in such nurturing activities when you may not be feeling like it, you will gain the benefits, even if you don't realise it at the time.

I found this to be an effective self-care strategy, as it can help to soothe and nourish the nervous system, help with any lower back pain or bodily aches after giving birth and through pregnancy itself.

I recommend avoiding the use of essential oils during pregnancy and breast-feeding, as the potency and hence the safety of the oil cannot be guaranteed. It can be much stronger and absorb through our skin and into our system very easily, especially when our skin is moist. It is advised not to be used on children under the age of two.

Coupled with some calming and healing frequency music or guided meditations, burning a beautiful candle with some grounding and relaxing scents, you will feel like you have had a beautiful warm hug. Make sure you have a support person around to check in on you regularly to make sure you do not fall asleep. Safety first given that you most likely will be tired!

GROUNDING ACTIVITIES AND SCENTS

The basis of Ayurveda is the philosophy of like increases like, so if when our *Vata dosha* is aggravated during childbirth, there is an aggravation of the elements of air and space. How can we balance this? Through utilising the elements of earth, water and fire as these provide the opposite effects and will work to balance this aggravation or imbalance known as *Vikruti*.

This is where 'grounding' practices are such valuable tools in relaxation and calming our nervous system. *Vata* aggravation presents with a stretching or over-stimulation of our nervous system and so enters our insomnia, anxiety, racing thoughts and depression.

It becomes vital then to add essences of earth, fire and water aspects in our lifestyle and practices, such as in the form of scents like *lavender, frankincense, chamomile, bergamot, neroli, rose, sandalwood, ylang ylang, myrrh and marjoram* as some examples of being effective tools.

Earthy tones as visuals in the brown, yellow and orange tones can bring about calm to the system. Steering away from the blacks and blues is a great idea when choosing flowers in the room, clothes to wear or imagery that you focus on.

Eating earthy, fiery and sweet foods and spices such as *sweet potato, pumpkin, cardamom, cinnamon, black pepper and ginger* as some very basic quick examples. Also heavier and moist foods such as ghee or porridge, rather than dry or light foods such as popcorn or processed type packaged foods, can be most nourishing to our body during this time.

We want to surround our whole home environment with earth elements utilising all of our senses of sight, smell, touch, taste and sounds. This will envelop our entire being with balance and to feel like a warm embrace.

Utilising plant and flower extracts for the smell can be very calming. It is a subtle healing tool that *combined* with medication, CBT, other psychologist tools, healing frequency music and a myriad of the other self-care strategies, can all have a cumulative effect in our recovery and well-being.

I am not claiming that a nice smell in a room will heal you of post-natal depression; not at all! However, I do believe that adding subtle aspects in the environment to have a cumulative effect, can alter *how* you feel whilst you are participating in Western treatment modalities. Sitting alone in my silent room was the *furthest* place of allowing healing, and if I had opened myself to changing the atmosphere and making little changes in how I felt, I feel like the suffering could have been so much less. Creating a softer environment for my *entire* family who were also trapped in my darkness, may have helped them too. Waiting for Western treatment to work is a reality of the situation, so having gentle tools to get us through that period is a missing link right now. One, that I certainly faced.

During my pregnancy I used to colour in mandalas with Ari and it was such a connective and creative activity that we did together. We would listen to music in the background, drink herbal teas together and it was a thing that we both looked forward to and enjoyed doing as a bonding activity. I felt like it completely supported my divine feminine mother aspect of myself. I felt so bountiful and nurturing whilst doing it, and carried this energy with me throughout the rest of the day.

I am working on creating mandalas with beautiful healing words, affirmations and focus phrases. My hope is that mothers can channel beautiful healing energies into creating these masterpieces, whilst directing their thoughts from darkness to absorbing the positive words on the page. I truly believe this can have an imprint on our subconscious and allow our hearts to open, as well as focus our anxious thoughts through this dark chapter into something more mindful. Ruminating on my loop didn't serve me. At all.

It requires us to remove the guilt of the time doing these 'useless or pointless' activities. Allowing ourselves to fully immerse in utilising the waiting time, into creative outlets in order to bring in pleasure and joy as well as focus into the mind.

Whilst I am not saying that colouring an affirmation-filled mandala will heal you...not at all! I am a strong advocate for Western medicine and treatment! It is simply a support tool that I wish I had utilised during my recovery journey, in the hope that it provides you and your family some respite too. Rather than sitting in my room alone, ruminating in my dark and spiralling thoughts, had I anchored into spending my energy into creative and deeply calming activities, then perhaps the journey may not have been crippled with so much pain. It may have been such a reconnecting activity to do with Ari, even silently knowing that we loved doing it before...I remember not knowing how to interact with him and going back to activities that we bonded in, could have helped *us* so much.

You deserve to be thriving. You deserve to feel amazing. You deserve to be back into your light and for the thick black fog to lift and dissipate.

Whilst taking the initiative and the reins into taking action, was not possible for me in the depths of my depression, as I was completely exhausted and engulfed by my darkness. However, if a path was laid out with tools that my husband could steer me through and create space for me to do, then I would have done them and my nervous system would have benefited without question.

ACCESS YOUR UNIQUE TOOL KIT OF RELAXATION STRATEGIES

This is a great time to reach into your tried and tested tool kit and utilise what makes *your* soul happy! We are all unique and feel relaxed and rejuvenated through different things. There was a recent post on Facebook that I loved which said, it is just as important to find your happiness triggers as it is knowing your triggers that make you feel bad.

I love to read, listen to Podcasts, listen to calm and relaxing frequency music or mantras, go for a walk along the water, take a nap and have a bath. I love to embrace my divine feminine and pamper myself with a nice blow-dry and manicure. Nothing refuels me more than sitting in a quiet space looking into nature or people-watching, as I have a coffee or a glass of wine. Sometimes it is just me doing literally nothing, as I watch the clouds and people pass on by.

We are all different and there is no right or wrong way of doing anything that you love! Find your pathway to bliss and NOW is the time to revel in these practices. Remove the guilt, shame and feeling like it is 'too indulgent' or like you do not have time with a newborn or baby. Appreciate the intrinsic value of *how* it will make you feel more 'normal' and help to restore your healing. I know that you may think taking care of dinner or the washing is pressing when you have a few more minutes up your sleeve. However, if you are not feeling well then you need to carve out space for your recovery and 'doing' one task after the next is not going to support your body, as much as 'being' and 'allowing' you to nourish and rejuvenate your body, mind and soul.

I shudder at how many hours I spent sitting in my room festering and suffocating in my thoughts. If someone had pulled me away and almost forced me to do different activities, it may have been a 'fake it until you make it' until I remembered what joy and spark these connective activities gave to me. All I know is that spending time in these activities would have been *so* much more beneficial to me and my family, than not doing anything at all.

I am a firm believer of doing activities with the intention of love and healing. In Ayurveda, it is said that adding feelings of guilt or shame can add to emotional *Ama* or emotional toxins, which is far more deleterious to our body than the act itself. Allow yourself the time and space to rejuvenate your body and connect with practices that used to bring you joy, so that this can bring you closer to feeling better. Allow your partner, family or friends to help steer you onto things that you love doing.

You may not feel like it at all but subtle energy shifts and reminders of how beautiful activities made you feel, will eventually feel joyous again. Though I am not a fan of the statement of 'fake it until you make it', in this case do the activities anyhow and in time the joy will return, but you will remain connected to the things you love rather than cut yourself off from everything, as I did.

8. REACH OUT TO A FRIEND OR FAMILY MEMBER TO TALK

If you are like me and get re-fuelled and revitalised by a beautiful soulful connection with someone, rather than sit in your room alone with your festering thoughts, I recommend reaching out to your beautiful sister, mother or a close friend and go for a coffee.

It may be difficult to organise; I understand how mammoth even simple tasks feel and how exhausting it may feel seeing someone. Yet, I remember after my toe surgery I had not been able to walk for more than 5 minutes at a time, until I was one-month post operation. I was asked to come out for a dinner with the mum's in Ari's class from school. I felt like I was in a bit of a funk, but I had so much fun! I felt invigorated and sparked back to life from connecting with people and just talking instead of being cooped up at home, made all the difference to bring me back to feeling amazing.

It was a gentle reminder for me that there is nothing quite like connecting with someone and you don't even need to talk about how you are feeling, if you don't want to. The very act of getting out of your house, seeing the sun and chatting about useless things, in and of itself can be so therapeutic. I would recommend doing it outdoors if possible, to soak in the sunshine and seeing how life is still rolling by around you, rather than a phone call...but I would still advocate for a phone call than doing nothing at all!

If you do feel like going out for dinner with a girlfriend or husband just to get out of the 'rut' and routine of Groundhog Day again and again, then do that! It is amazing what a little change in energy can bring about to how you feel and what levels of optimism and hope that you have for life itself, when you see that life is still happening around you.

9. DO SOMETHING THAT YOU NORMALLY LOVE TO DO THAT SPARKS YOU UP

This is the time to go into your toolbox of what you know sparks your heart and soul. Allow yourself the time and space to delve into it full force! The spark and zest for life may be rekindled within you when doing this activity, which ultimately is so therapeutic and healing for you.

I absolutely love to go for a walk along the water and this reminds me of how expansive the universe and all of nature is, and how small my problems are in comparison to the enormity of life. It allows me to put things into perspective and I always feel more calm and connected to life when I do this.

Since I was not able to make a decisive action step of driving to the beach and doing this, it would be up to my husband to make this happen, knowing how much I loved it. The sun on my skin, the wind in my hair and the ocean in my toes would have an impact in removing some of that helplessness and perhaps allow me to feel a little more connected to life. If I did this whilst holding my baby in my Baby Bjorn, then what an even more connective experience this would be and what a better use of time, rather than sitting in my room ruminating and hoping that something would change!

10. TURN OFF THE TV AND UNNECESSARY NOISE OR
    STIMULATION
When we understand that our nervous systems need to be soothed, nourished and rejuvenated, this forms the basis of all of my strategies to assist in your healing. I personally struggled with the stimuli and intensity of the T.V. The noise, erratic sounds and volume intonations absolutely aggravated my *Vata dosha* imbalance, that was present after childbirth. It was akin to hearing nails on a chalkboard for me and I simply needed a calm and peaceful environment in every aspect.

I especially found the news very heavy and added to my feelings of anxiety, so I would need it turned off. I would also suggest turning off any other stimulation that may be adding to your anxiety, including social media. I have mentioned social media quite a bit, but more so because it can stimulate so many triggers within us, that if it is causing a reaction within you, whether it be the constant feed, certain groups or certain people, then 'unfollow' or switch it off.

11. SUPPORT YOURSELF WITH AS MUCH SLEEP AS POSSIBLE
Similar to the strategy to minimise stress, this too may sound as foreign a concept with a newborn! I did struggle with the phrase 'sleep when the baby sleeps' as our boys had major sleep issues until they were six months old. I literally could have thrown a brick at someone every time they said that!

Yet, our biology requires us to have a minimum of six to eight hours of uninterrupted, good quality sleep so that our systems can re-calibrate, rest and recover for healthy functioning of all of our systems. They say that an average parent loses up to 109 minutes of sleep every night for the first year after having a baby. They also say that an average of 6-months' worth of sleep is lost within the first two-years of the baby's life. There is sleep debt that accrues and this can have serious impacts on our health and well-being.

Couple this data with your possible inability to fall asleep even if your baby is sleeping, as was the case with me for almost the entire 11 weeks...it is no wonder you feel tired! The sleep debt that ensued from that, together with my baby boys that woke a good 7 to 8 times a night and napped for no longer than 40 minutes at a time, until we hit the six-month mark, was *exhausting* and I daresay so taxing to my body. The body requires sleep and there is no shortcut around this.

So what is my advice? I would say that if you have a partner or husband that can help you with some of the night feeds so you can have a solid stint of sleep, then accept it! If they are working through the week, then ask and allow them to do it over the weekend, as it is not humanly possible or fair to be honest, to shoulder all of the night feeds yourself. This can build harbouring resentment and hostility within your relationship, as you may not feel as if there is an equal sharing of the parenting tasks. Being open and transparent with your needs as a human, is essential to get the best support that you need and deserve!

If you can nap whilst the baby sleeps then do that. If your partner or family member can come sit with the baby whilst you catch up on sleep, then ask and accept it. It is vital to prioritise sleep and remove the guilt or shame in asking, and completely revel in the knowledge that sleep is a basic human requirement. It is *not* selfish in asking for help so that you get your much needed sleep. It is a vital part of your healing.

If, like me, you cannot sleep even when given countless opportunities and support, speak to your physician to get some medical treatment just for a short time to help support this biological need. It works by breaking the cycle and restoring your body's natural circadian rhythm as best as possible with a newborn. They can provide medications or supplements with safety, based on your medical history, your presenting symptoms, other medications you are taking and whether or not you are pregnant or breastfeeding. It is important to discuss options with a doctor and/or pharmacist before self-selecting anything over-the-counter.

It is an important part of healing so be open and honest with what physical and mental symptoms you are having, so they can best target your treatment to optimise your healing. I too struggled even whilst trying different sleep aids, and perhaps the stress of that added to my anxiety which then caused even more sleep issues! Fun times! However, I am proud of myself for being open about what symptoms I had and took action accordingly, irrespective of the outcome.

Because sleep is so important for you and your baby, I have been working with Listening to Smile to create healing frequency tracks with binaural beats, to help support sleep for both of you. I saw first-hand that I needed support tools to enable me to sleep, but had no access to them and felt so frustrated when I was told to sleep, but nothing I tried worked!

The healing music with the appropriate frequencies may assist the mind and body to bring on sleep, by exerting a calming effect. They are carefully curated tracks with subtle subconscious messages of connection, healing and self-love affirmations to again allow healing at a cellular level, in an almost (but not actual) hypnosis modality. It brings you and your baby's soul, the message of love and connection, to help fill this void that post-natal depression can bring. The tone brings about calming, grounding and healing in order to help induce and encourage sleep. Make sleep your priority and remember, that you are deserving of this basic human right, irrespective of the fact that you have just had a baby.

Whilst it isn't recommended to 'teach' self-settling techniques for sleep until your baby is 6-months old, not sleeping for 6 months isn't necessarily the most sustainable or viable option! I do then advocate for utilising services or programs to help your baby whether it be through Tresillian, Karitane or other outreach programs. These are available upon a referral from your GP, so it's definitely worth discussing your baby's sleep with them. They can be truly life-saving and repair the strain in families, though I am mindful that embarking upon this type of journey can be anxiety provoking in and of itself. I also appreciate that self-settling techniques may be considered very harsh and cruel for a young baby, so I appreciate all sides of the coin here!

Irrespective of where you stand on this, I want to give you hope that sleep deprivation will *not* last forever and there will be light at the end of the tunnel. I remember thinking with Ari that this would be my life *forever* and I resented motherhood for that, as I love my sleep! Yet, at six months when I did sleep train him in his own room, despite some ebbs and flows through teething or developmental leaps, he slept through the night and I could walk out of the room and he would self-soothe and sleep all through the night. Life changing! Hang in there as it will not be forever, unless you have young children back to back then perhaps yes, your broken sleep will be longer than my experience.

There are strategies that you can try to assist you with your sleep. They are referred to as 'sleep hygiene' strategies. Whilst it may be a matter of trial and error to find what exactly works for you, it would be worth a try if your eyeballs are hanging out of your head. They can be utilised at any time in your life to assist in good quality sleep!

1. Turn off the T.V, phone and all devices at least 1 hour before you want to go to sleep, to avoid the blue-light and unnecessary stimulation. There are blue-light blocking glasses that can minimise the impact that this light causes within our system throughout the day. This light can affect the production of melatonin, which is responsible for our

circadian rhythm required for natural sleep cycles. Visit the *Sleep Health Foundation* for some amazing information about this.

2. Exercise during the day, but not within 90-minutes of bedtime as it can work to arouse you too close to bedtime. Through the day, exercise will encourage good quality sleep.

3. Try to have an oil massage with warmed sesame oil, to calm the nervous system and pacify the aggravated *Vata dosha*. If a full body massage feels too overwhelming, then at least apply the warm oil to the crown of your head, gently and minimally in/on your ears and on the soles of your feet. Then, followed by a warm bath with plant and flower essences, as well as magnesium as a muscle relaxant. Soothing the nervous system, particularly at night may help to induce sleep.

4. Stay away from caffeine in tea, coffee and chocolate before sleeping, and for some you may need to abstain as early as midday. Trial and error is the best way to work out what time should be the latest that you consume it. For me it is 4pm at the latest, whilst recent studies suggest 2pm is the ideal 'cut-off' time.

5. Be mindful of eating very heavy, oily or fried food as it may cause heartburn and indigestion. Try not eating within 2-hours of bedtime, as lying down can impede digestion and alter the quality or ability to sleep. Sleeping with more raised or 'propped up' pillows may help with gravity for digestion, if you are finding that a heavy meal is affecting your capacity to sleep well.

6. Try a guided meditation to help you redirect your thoughts and calm the mind.

7. Essential oils can have queries in regards to their safety, due to their potency for use during pregnancy and in small children under two. If you are pregnant or breastfeeding or have your baby in the same room, then I would recommend you use natural plant essence infusion types but utilising *lavender, frankincense, chamomile, bergamot, neroli, rose, sandalwood, ylang ylang, myrrh and marjoram.* These gentler essences are examples for use, as they can help to promote or enhance relaxation and support sleep.

8. Keep the room dark and use an eye-mask if there is light in the room. Some people find benefit in a weighted eye mask or a weighted/heavy blanket in reducing anxiety and calming the nervous system. Use ear-plugs if outside noise is causing any disruption.

9. Journal or write down any constant or intrusive thoughts, so that it is cleared from your mind before going to sleep.

10. Have a herbal tea, but not with too much liquid so that you do not need to use the bathroom throughout the night. Think of *chamomile, lemon balm, passionflower or lavender.* Even boiled milk with some turmeric, cacao, ghee, cinnamon and/or cardamom with a touch of honey at the end, can also soothe the nervous system and calm the body to promote sleep; again not too much liquid to wake you up for the bathroom.

11. Deep breathing can help to relax the nervous system and calm the whole body down.

12. Do not do any other activity in bed other than sleep or intimacy, so that your body connects the bed to sleep and not eating or watching T.V. It becomes your sanctuary for sleep.

12. AYURVEDIC FOOD, AYURVEDIC TEAS AND HERBS/SPICES
Ayurveda has allowed me to have a true appreciation for the honouring, rejuvenation and nourishment of mothers through their ancient practices and philosophies. Ironically, I perceived them to be very much old-wives' tales growing up, and did not have the capacity for true appreciation until delving into my own formal education.

The principle of like increases like, is a firm foundation of Ayurveda and *Vata* aggravation post-delivery causes the excess of air and space elements within our bodies. This can be balanced through utilising the opposing elements of fire, earth and water.

We also want to bring about the opposing qualities of the *vata dosha* (cold, mobile, dry, light, subtle, rough, clear) which are namely; hot, moist, heavy, oily, stable, smooth, dense and sticky/not clear. These properties that we bring in the form of spices, food, teas and practices work to restore balance within our vitiated system.

It is through the mindful eating of Ayurvedic perspective foods, that can help to support a mother's recovery, particularly in this 'fourth trimester' after birth. It forms to nourish and rejuvenate the system and adds warmth and grounding. Rather than fast-food or even frozen foods, that hold little to no *Prana* or life-force, we want to encourage the eating of fresh Ayurvedic principled prepared foods.

If you can subscribe to a freshly prepared meal service or if your community arranges one, then say yes! If your family or friends bring you home-made meals, then welcome the love and beautiful intention that is immersed in that cooking. It will work to nourish your body, mind and soul. Welcome it with open arms and gratitude, and choose *prana* filled food wherever you can.

To help this process of nutrition a little easier to access, I am creating an Ayurvedic cook book together with a tea range. These are all centred around reducing your *Vata* aggravation and to bring about balance and healing. If we utilise food, spices, tea as rejuvenating tools, then our nourishment becomes incorporated at *least* three to five times a day, which is very significant and impactful!

If your family and/or partner can freshly prepare these with a beautiful, mindful and soulful feeling infused into them, then the food will become medicinal in and of itself. Beautiful heart-centred intentions in the cooking, will energetically infuse into the food and in Ayurveda we refer to this as the *Sadhana* of the kitchen. This is the mindful and conscious food preparation within the kitchen space, to essentially create high vibrational food that will most optimise the body's health and well-being. This can be done by a prayer whilst cooking, reciting a mantra or filling your heart and mind with thoughts and intentions of infusing the food with love and healing.

I also love saying a prayer before we eat our food, so that we are infusing our mind and body with so much gratitude for the beautiful food that is about to nourish our bodies. We thank all of the people involved in allowing this meal to be possible, and fill our hearts with gratitude that we have food in our bodies to help fuel and rejuvenate us. I have a beautiful mandala that I coloured in with Ari, that has our prayer written on it that we utilise even today.

It is a beautiful ritual and begins the eating process with pure mindfulness and gratitude. It also sets our eating practices to be conscious, and aiding our digestion and assimilation of the nutrients into every cell of our body. This is very contrasting to eating whilst driving or on the run.

13. AYURVEDIC PRACTICES

I have learned that the aim of post-natal care for the mother, is designed in supporting her body, mind and spirit to heal and rejuvenate after delivering her baby and to pacify or reduce the *Vata* aggravation that biologically ensues after delivery.

As explained above, we want to bring on practices that are heating, oily, heavy (think grounding), smooth, sticky and dense.

Enter forth *Abhyanga* or the practice of self-massage, or if your partner or family member can massage your body for you. Ayurveda states that cold pressed sesame oil that is slightly warmed, provides the oleation and warmth that our body needs, when there is *Vata* aggravation. The oil will nourish, soothe and relax the nervous system and pacify the aggravated *Vata*, which presents with erratic and fast thoughts, insomnia, anxiety and depression.

To support women in utilising this modality to nourish the nervous system, I am in the process of creating Ayurvedic massage oils to allow you to get the most out of this practice. It will guide you on how to massage your head, body and what to do before, during and afterwards so that it works to nourish your nervous system and bring your body back into balance and best support you on your journey to recovery, whilst utilising Western treatments.

Utilising the benefits of warmth, oleation or moisturising, as well as certain essences to help bring upon relaxation through the skin, can assist in grounding your *Vata* aggravation. I would also advise on keeping your body warm, not exposed to too much wind or stimuli during this healing time and especially in this fourth trimester as your body comes back into equilibrium.

Ayurveda also looks at being mindful with all of the lifestyle choices that are taken in through all of our five senses, as they have an impact on our mind, body and soul. Listening to very loud and aggressive type music or watching fighting movies for example, can affect the quality of the mind. It can affect the *gunas* or attributes of the mind from being *sattwic* (pure, centred, peaceful), *rajasic* (intense, consumed, stimulated, busy) or *tamasic* (inert, dull, unmotivated).

If we make conscious choices in all that we take in through our senses, then the quality of our mind can be enhanced. This will allow for us to live a life with a greater connection to our body and spirit. This in turn, allows for more clarity to continuously make positive choices for ourselves. It is a very empowering modality that encourages mindfulness, and to make positive choices that support our well-being.

14. INFANT MASSAGE

Learning how to give your baby a massage is also an amazing part of your healing. Through touch, it can enhance your bonding and attachment with your baby.

It also works to enhance serotonin and dopamine for better mood, oxytocin which is the 'love hormone' for relaxation and connection, and it enhances melatonin to assist with sleep for both you and your baby. Massage also reduces cortisol, which is your stress hormone. This hormone reduction can work to get you out of the 'fight or flight' way of being. It can help therefore, to reduce symptoms of anxiety and depression as well as help with insomnia, which are all amazing changes to our biochemistry, that undeniably can make a difference to the way that we feel. I certainly would have welcomed even a slight change to my biochemistry, to allow me to feel even once micro-millimetre better.

It is undeniable that learning how to massage your baby is a beautiful practice to incorporate into your day as you heal. I wish with all of my heart, that I had known this whilst I was in the throes of my post-natal depression, when I stayed away from my boys except to do what was required. My heart breaks as to not knowing that there was this amazing tool available, that would have supported *both* of our healing, rather than locking myself in a quiet and sterile room ruminating over my dark thoughts. An experience that facilitates closeness and connection, is one that is *undeniably* necessary, when disconnection to your baby or children is a symptom of your post-natal depression.

This excites me so much as to spreading the importance of this practice in the recovery for women with post-natal depression. It is such a wonderful and practical tool to help with the bonding and attachment to our baby in the most significant way, which is a particularly relevant symptom of PND. My hope, is that I can teach health professionals the importance of this tool with my Paediatric Massage Consultant (PMC) training, as well as teach as many mothers as possible how to massage their babies with my CIMI (Certified Infant Massage Instructor) qualifications. I would love for this gentle modality to form an essential tool, to help the bonding and attachment for our mothers; which is the cruelest symptom of PND, that still rips my heart out even today.

15. CREATE A CONDUCIVE ENVIRONMENT FOR HEALING
In a similar tangent to what I was explaining above, I do believe in creating the environment so that it is conducive to healing through our five senses;

    i.   smells through diffusers, incense or candles
    ii.   sound through music and mantras
    iii.   sight through beautiful imagery or seeing nature
    iv.   touch through massage or feeling the grass/nature
    v.   taste through utilising the *Vata* grounding herbs, tastes and spices

Go out in nature as much as you possibly can. Not just to tend to errands or the groceries, but to fully immerse yourself within nature and being mindfully present! Cover your ears with a beanie if it is windy or cold, keep warm but go for walks outside and breathe in the fresh air deeply and mindfully. Touch the grass with your feet and if you are lucky to be near an ocean or river, then listen closely to the sound, and walk in the water as long as it isn't freezing cold... and I am aware that I sound like an Indian Aunty with my advice of keeping warm!

I often light incense or clear my house with a sage stick, to cleanse the energies especially after an argument or frustration energy with my boys! Whilst I do not have clinical trial data to tell you how effective, if at all it may be, I personally just feel better through the ritual and there is nothing like a ceremonial re-set to change the atmosphere that is around us.

Open up the windows to let in fresh air and keep your house as bright through the day as you possibly can. I thrive on light! It is so deeply nourishing and energetically clearing for the space that you are in. Our apartment in Cairns was extremely dark. Ari and I matched that dark energy in that space, to the dark fog that I felt at the time. When I had recovered I could not stay in that apartment, as it just energetically traumatised me to remembering my time being ill there.

Our home in Perth had a double void with beautiful light coming through. Whilst I had PND in that home too, I had no change in how I felt there because the light and cleansing effect that it had, made me feel like it shone even brighter when I had recovered. Natural sunlight is very underrated! Open your blinds and windows and bask in the beauty that nature has given to us for free!

I also had trouble making any decisions AT ALL, so deciding what to wear would take me an unnecessarily long time. Yet, I would say there is so much benefit and importance to having a shower or bath every day and putting on a fresh pair of clothes. Ask your partner to help you have a shower and lay an outfit out for you, if you cannot physically do it. I would say the energetic washing away of that stagnant and dark energy, will have an impact on how you feel and slowly bring you back into routine and feeling better about yourself. The *waterfall meditation* further along in the book, is a good practice to try in the shower too to cleanse away stagnant energy and feelings. Imagine the wordings as you have a shower and feel the energies washing away from your body.

As much as you possibly can, try to do one beautiful act of self-care that you used to love doing. I wrote earlier about how it is just as important to know your happiness triggers, as it is your unhappy triggers. Now is the time to lean on what you already know makes you feel good. You may not feel like it and it may feel so hard, and possibly luxurious or selfish, but NOW is the time to take steps towards what makes you feel good and walk towards that.

16. STOP WORRYING ABOUT OTHERS
Do not compare. Do not worry about the impact your PND is having on others. Do not worry about other people's judgement or thoughts. Do not worry about what your neighbours may think of you or the crying baby. None of this is important right now.

I hand on my heart can say that unless you have experienced post-natal depression first hand, then no one else can understand exactly what you are going through. Any comments they may make such as 'snap out of it', 'it could be worse', 'be thankful for all that you have' etc. are not statements that come from a place of understanding. Therefore, do not make yourself feel bad for something that someone else cannot understand.

Remove any feelings of guilt and shame and redirect them into activities that are positive and conducive to your healing. Right now, you only need to think about yourself and getting better as best you can, so that you can be *fully* available for your family and baby.

You are *not* a burden on others and you are trying your best to recover and heal from a condition, that does not have a black and white cause, solution or reason for you. The weight of others can be set down, as well as all the other unnecessary baggage that you may be carrying. You no *longer* need to worry about carrying that load and focus on your recovery, so that your life can return to its glory as you and your entire family deserve.

17. BE GENTLE ON YOURSELF

Be kind to yourself and do not berate yourself for your mind and body not functioning the way you would like them to, or the way you assume others are functioning. Shower your body and mind with compassion and forgiveness. Remove every inch of resentment and frustration that you may be carrying.

I say that, because I felt like my body had ripped me off and taken away the most precious time with the early bonding with my newborn. I felt extremely betrayed and had to work through a lot of healing and forgiveness to my body, for experiencing it twice. What I realised is that, harbouring these feelings served no purpose for anybody, made me end up feeling worse and flooded my body with more anger and cortisol than it already needed! What would it change?

Body image is a sensitive topic for all mothers of a newborn. No matter how much or little weight one gained during pregnancy, there is no doubt feelings of shock or sadness present towards our changing body. Some may be filled with complete awe and amazement, as to what our bodies can create and give birth to. That is a beautifully healthy and empowering way to feel. I felt like I was not prepared for the changes in my physical body, but certainly had more understanding and compassion the second time round.

Imagine, if we *thanked* our bodies for growing a beautiful baby deep within our wombs and for carrying them out into this big world?

Imagine, if we *thanked* our bodies for changing the way it needed to house and birth our babies? Imagine, if we *thanked* our bodies for nourishing our babies in utero and now through our breast milk?

How empowering and *liberating* this self-talk is, instead of berating ourselves for not 'bouncing' back to our twenty-year old selves?

How much lighter and forgiving is this tone, rather than making ourselves feel bad for not looking like the celebrities on the front cover of magazines or plastered all over social media?

Being harsh, mean and critical serves no purpose other than to make us feel worse about ourselves, and I don't know what good could ever come out of it. We need to treat ourselves with the same respect, admiration and kindness that we would to our children or sister. We need to look at ourselves in the mirror, with our warts and all, and acknowledge what bountiful, beautiful and amazing creators and beings we are. If we never forgot the inner knowing, that we are the divine within, then we would never speak to ourselves with such cruelty.

Choose loving words to yourself. Choose kindness and compassion. Always x

18. GRATITUDE

There is a saying, 'to live by the attitude of gratitude' and there is merit to the saying. Though, I was unable to see anything positive or amazing about most things when I was in the thick of it, I wonder in retrospect what altering my inner conversation from one of being dark, stuck and unable to think properly, to one of gratitude. What might that have done to my inner well-being?

I remember family members and my GP telling me that I had so much to be grateful for, and at the time I wanted to scream when they said that! I felt like they didn't understand what I was feeling, that my head was in a vacant fog and that it seemed like a very easy thing to do...and not actually possible to execute with how I was feeling.

Yet, the truth was, I did have *so* much I could still focus on being grateful for. Grateful, for having a roof over our heads and that my husband and family could help me with everything involved with having a newborn and running the entire household. Grateful, for having healthy children and my own physically healthy body. Grateful, that I found the right access to health care that I needed and for having so many beautiful Earth angels to carry me through my journey.

If we can focus our attention on what greatness we do have, instead of focussing on all the things that may not be ideal, then we become *more* aware of things to be grateful for, and it is very addictive. Infusing our bodies with endorphins will have a profound impact on the way we feel, which can in turn make us more grateful! It may be a matter of faking it until you make, it and whilst ordinarily I dislike that statement a lot, in this instance it may be enough to shift your mindset into one of optimism and hope.

First thing in the morning, think of the first three things you are grateful for. Repeat the same before you go to bed at night. Every time your thoughts go into a negative spiral, think of one different thing to be grateful for and repeat it as many times as you catch yourself spiralling.

You may well find that inherently your thoughts may navigate from being very heavy, to ones filled with gratitude. It would be a beautiful bonding activity to do with your partner as well as with your older child, as a way of shifting the energy and filling everyone with optimism by embracing the present and being hopeful for a beautiful future ahead.

As a family we have a ritual where we each say three things that we are thankful for, before the boys hop into bed after their bath. It is a ritual that I love doing and even Ruphus gets a turn. Though, the boys normally do it for him by saying 'woof' and we all have a good giggle! Laughter is also another tool to cash in on when you can!

19. GO OUT IN NATURE, BREAK UP THE DAILY ROUTINE
I have described the importance of going out in nature a lot, as the effects of the beautiful sunshine, fresh air and immersing yourself in nature is so healing. It allows you to feel the expansive nature of life. For me, it helps me place my feelings and problems in perspective, when I get so caught up into thinking that my issues are all-encompassing.

I thrive on routine and predictability, but there is nothing quite like breaking up a monotonous routine, to add some vigour and spark to your days. I found that life became quite Groundhog Day in nature so to go for a walk somewhere new or going to a new café, can be very helpful. Lockdown with Covid also highlights the importance of breaking up the daily routine, to give the concept of time changing and not stuck in the boring 'same old' thing day after day.

HEALTH TIP:

SLEEP HYGIENE STRATEGIES

These are some sleep strategies that can assist you in getting to sleep and promoting good quality sleep;

+ Ideally do not eat large meals within 2 hours of sleeping, as it can disrupt sleep

+ Avoid or at least minimise alcohol. It may induce sleep but it can disrupt the quality of it

+ Avoid caffeine in tea, coffee, chocolate from early afternoon; even midday for some people

+ Spend 30 minutes winding down before trying to go to sleep

+ Dim your lighting, turn off the T.V and phone to minimise the effects from blue light

+ Ideally no devices for 1 hour before bed, as it can cause overstimulation for the nervous system

+ Try relaxation activities such as a warm bath, herbal teas (not too much liquid), reading

+ Write a list of things on your mind, so that it is cleared from your mind and put aside

+ No vigorous exercise within 90 minutes of sleep, as it can keep you in an alert and hyperactive state

CHAPTER 8

TOOLS FOR THE PARTNER AND FAMILY/CARER

M y *whole* family felt the strain that my illness caused. My husband, my children, Ruphus our fur-baby, my parents, in-laws, our siblings and their partners. We are very blessed that we have family and they supported us as much as possible every moment and every step of the way. For that we are eternally grateful. I feel sad that I burdened *all* of them with my recovery and whilst it was not intentional, nor was I aware at the time of just how strong my hold was on them, the level of stress and worry that I imparted onto them; I am *profusely* sorry that it had such a grasping and rippling effect.

It is completely natural for there to be different dynamics within a family unit. Personalities and views on a situation may not be seen through the same filter during a crisis as stressful and all-encompassing as this. There can be perhaps multiple opinions or thoughts as to how things should be done, all coming from their own level of understanding, experience and lens through which they view life and situations. Knowing this, can hopefully impart some respite into how you feel about your current situation.

However, the added tension and unnecessary strain from any differing methodologies and perspectives, *can* compound the already delicate situation. I believe that everyone should work for the common good of the patient; no more and no less. *She* needs to be held in the forefront and in everyone's mind's eye at all times, with all conversations and decisions that are made.

I believe that what is required and best for the mother, is for cohesion and a synergistic collaborative approach from all family and friends, in all dealings with her and the situation. It comes from the perspective that open communication is vital and the patient *must* be the centre of everyone's focus. The intention behind all activities and conversations, needs to be centred around what will benefit *her* the most. Idealistic possibly, but oh so important.

Working together towards the same common goal in a calm and collective manner, must be the *only* priority for all involved. Stripping away the extra noise that takes away from her focus in getting better, is so important. Lighten her load. Let her place any additional baggage down off her shoulders and heart, so that walking towards her healing and recovery, is less heavy and difficult than she needs it to be.

These points are relevant for those who are lucky enough *to* have family who care, are available and are there to support you in this journey. What a blessing! There are so many women that do not have family or friends around them to give support, and this adds a *whole* new element of pressure and strain of not having anyone to lean on. In this instance, it becomes very important to find the support that you need to hold on. Whether it is friends, your neighbour, someone who you meet in your community, mothers group or school...speak up and reach out. You are needing support, and you will be amazed as to how beautiful people can rise up to the occasion to look after you. It is a beautiful opportunity to see the goodness in people, because there is no need to venture through each day alone. Some of those mothers and families, may have been through the same torture.

The way out of how I was feeling, of feeling like I was drowning, suffocating, couldn't breathe and feeling like there was no hope or future for me; was unequivocally using my husband and family as a raft, a lifeline to hold on to. Sometimes I would speak to the ones in my home or call the ones not at home, every half an hour to get me through to the next hour...sometimes I would be on the phone to them all day despite them all having their own jobs, children and life to contend with. I sunk my claws and clutches into all of them; one at a time, just like holding onto a life raft in the ocean putting all my weight onto them, hoping that I wouldn't drown.

They *all* held me up and kept me taking my breaths of life, one at a time. They gave me the space and *allowed* me to express my feelings and thoughts, one at a time. They gave me the space to let it all hang out.

Below I have listed some tools and some reflections that may help another partner and family/carer, to help navigate through this time with a little more ease and grace, so that you *also* do not feel alone within this stressful chapter. I *completely* acknowledge what you are going through and how you would be feeling, as well as carrying the weight of the world on your shoulders. It is so important for you to look after yourself as well, so that you don't drown by being her life raft. It can *so* easily happen, so now is the time to not forget about you and all that you are doing for her during this time.

Thank you for being there for her and never giving up on her x

She needs you and whilst she may not be able to articulate it right now; she is so utterly grateful for you standing by her, standing up for her and being her voice when she has lost her way. Your piece in the puzzle of her recovery, is so important and deserves to be celebrated!

Thank you! Thank you! Thank you!

Just keep the vision of her healing and recovering from this in your mind's eye and hold her in the forefront of each and every day. *Never give up faith or hope and take the time to look after your needs as well, and you will ALL survive this time, I* promise!

SUMMARY OF TOOLS FOR THE PARTNER AND FAMILY/CARER

1. Be honest with others as to what is happening and allow help
2. Healthy and Prana/life-force rich food is vital during this time
3. Talk to a good friend or support person to vent
4. Take action for your partner
5. Take time off work if possible
6. Nurture your older child that may feel so lost and confused
7. Mindfulness strategies
8. Exercise
9. No blame game
10. Open communication and allow space for healing within your relationship
11. Seven unhelpful things as a carer to say or do

TOOL 1: BE HONEST WITH OTHERS AS TO WHAT IS HAPPENING AND ALLOW HELP

I do strongly believe that unless you have experienced post-natal depression before, have seen it first-hand or are reading more about it, then there is no way to fully appreciate the depths of what the situation is. If you have not seen mental health conditions before, then this may feel extremely foreign and scary.

How can one explain this to friends without kids? With kids with a healthy mother? If they haven't gone through it, it can be so hard to explain the darkness that entrenches the entire space; what was a home with so many feelings of love, joy, optimism and hope has lost all meaning. Now all that is remaining is a space filled with darkness, fear, guilt and shame.

By constantly raising awareness that life after having a baby is not always rainbows and butterflies, I hope this makes it easier for you to speak out. If we talk about it more and raise awareness, then the guilt and shame around asking for help absolves and we can ask for help as easily as we would after we had a knee operation. With understanding comes compassion and true empathy.

Delegate what you can to family or friends and don't be afraid or embarrassed to ask for help. We were *so* lucky that we had family with us from interstate, otherwise we would have sunk like a huge ship going through this alone. Hands down. There was *no* way to look after the household, our businesses, child/children, and dog, all the while with the anchor of the house down and out.

Get family and friends to help with the groceries, playdates for the older child, school drop off and pickups, cooking, cleaning...you name it; if you feel like you need help doing it, then ask.

TOOL 2: HEALTHY AND PRANA RICH/LIFE-FORCE RICH FOOD IS VITAL DURING THIS TIME

Food preparation is a very healing part of the post-natal journey where consuming warm, moist, oily, heavy foods filled with *prana* (life-force and energy) and beautiful nutrients, will help to rejuvenate the mother *and* the *whole family* as well. Utilising

Ayurvedic principles of meals, teas, spices and herbs can help to support *all* of your bodies during this stressful time, especially in the first 40 days as they will all help to balance this aggravated system that naturally happens with a new baby in the home.

If you are able to cook or delegate *freshly* prepared meals to your family or friends to bring to you, then invest in an Ayurvedic recipe book to help you create the best meals for post-natal care. They will be designed with the most appropriately selected ingredients and spices to nourish your bodies and allow the food to become rejuvenating in and of itself.

The principles can be applied to any food type, style or taste so that everyone can benefit from balancing the aggravated *Vata dosha,* which occurs after birth as well as in a busy, hustle-bustle lifestyle with disrupted sleep and erratic routines when a new baby comes home. It is not only Indian food that it can prepare, but the principles applied to *all* food preparation and tastes, is what exerts their balancing effects within the system.

If you are unable to cook daily then try to sign up for a meal delivery service with home cooked or freshly prepared meals, or sign up to a meal train within your community.

I would recommend limiting greasy takeaway convenience food, processed foods, excessive alcohol and caffeine. *Prana* (life-force) rich food from fresh produce (ideally organic) or sourced from a farmer's market, will have the most nutrient dense qualities. If we add cloudy and non-nutrient rich foods, then the clarity of our minds gets affected, which in turn can affect our reactions and the way we cope with situations. We want clean, nutrient dense and high vibration foods prepared and eaten with love, so that it becomes therapeutic and ensures a clear state of mind.

Dull, processed, stale, leftovers, excessive alcohol/caffeine and nutrient lacking foods can affect the mind to become *rajasic* (agitated, active, aggressive) or *tamasic* (dull, inert, unmotivated) in quality. This is opposite to the sattwic (calm, serene, composed and clear) quality of mind, that would allow you to handle the stress with poise and clarity that it needs.

If you are having your tribe help you with food, try to minimise the disruption of delivery and returning the containers to reduce the logistics that the newly birthed mother has to think about. Help is best when it is seamless, action-based and not too heavy with planning, as it can strip energy away from the mother who solely needs to focus on her healing. This is a good opportunity to say, that as friends or carers, instead of asking the mother to reach out if she needs anything, make a solid offering that she can accept rather than her needing to ask for help. That 'reaching IN' vs her having to 'reach OUT', can be a gesture of truly being there for her.

+ Make sure you stay hydrated with at least 8 to 10 glasses of room temperature or warm water each day (icy cold water can reduce the digestive fire from an Ayurvedic perspective)

+ Limit the amount of caffeine, which can stimulate your nervous system and add anxiety and irritability to how you are feeling, as well as disrupt your natural sleep rhythms

+ Limit alcohol to a minimal level, so that it does not act as a depressant within your system and cloud your ability to help your partner through this dark time

TOOL 3: TALK TO A GOOD FRIEND OR SUPPORT PERSON TO VENT

It is also vital for the support people to have someone that they can trust and talk to about what is happening. It is healthy to vent and talk about your concerns and feelings, otherwise it can become like a pressure cooker waiting to erupt.

As a member of the family or friend, reach out and be there for the partner and family who most likely are crippled with fear as to what is going on. They would feel like they will be stuck in this situation forever, and this can be a very hard concept to wrap their head around, as to when that light will return.

Go out for a coffee or drink, go for a walk together or simply pick up the phone and engage in conversation with someone neutral, who can just be there to listen and support you.

I would highly recommend making sure the mother has someone that can stay with her, to make sure she is safe and looked after at that time, if it is at a very serious level. You will then have peace of mind, as you unplug for a little while.

A problem shared is a problem halved, and the advice you receive may be exactly what you need to hear.

TOOL 4: TAKE ACTION FOR YOUR PARTNER

If you suspect that your partner or family member has post-natal depression, then speak up for her if she is unable to recognise it within herself. Be the eyes, ears and voice to seek the help from her obstetrician, GP or child health nurse, rather than being in denial or hoping that it will get better on its own. She may well convince you that she is fine, but if deep within your bones you know that not to be true, then now is the time to hold her hand when she needs it the most.

Health professionals can arrange for a mental health plan (ask for a long appointment to do this properly); which now with Covid includes 20 bulk-billed sessions to a psychologist. I would ask to be referred to perinatal specific doctors, as this is their bread and butter.

I personally struggled with being able to find doctors with my cognition and not being able to concentrate, that I needed someone to take the reins and guide me to the help.

Post-natal depression is characterised by having symptoms lasting for _at least two weeks_, so let this time frame be your gauge into knowing when to access help. Be the strength and voice that she needs to access treatment as the longer it is left, the deeper or worse the situation can become.

TOOL 5: TAKE TIME OFF WORK IF POSSIBLE

If possible I would advise to take time off work, for as long as you possibly can financially. Whilst it seems like there is no light at the end of tunnel, the sooner she gets treatment and care, that light will return sooner. Waiting will not help the situation get better. I know there is fear of job security, the reality of life and bills etc. but without proper attention and care, this situation could last for much longer or get much worse.

I hope that this becomes mainstream knowledge so that bosses will be more attentive and attuned to the realities for some households after having a baby. I hope that they can show you kindness, empathy and patience with arms wide open.

If you work for a company and can help that person, then help. If you can delay their bills by a month or 6 weeks, then lend an olive branch so these families can access the help they need at a time that they need it most.

TOOL 6: NURTURE YOUR OLDER CHILD THAT MAY FEEL SO LOST AND CONFUSED

If you have older children as we did the second time around, there is an extra responsibility to look after this poor older child. Ari was only 4-years old at the time of my second baby's arrival, and he would have felt so lost, scared and confused as to what was unfolding. It showed in the form of anger, frustration and a huge disconnection from me and it all transpired overnight for him.

They would blame the baby for this chaos or just not be able to process the heaviness of what is happening, in their once happy home. Their whole world would have been turned upside down and this can be so abrupt in setting as it was for me, that how on earth could a 4-year-old understand this?

It was because of this turmoil for poor Ari, that I wrote my children's book '_My Mummy After Our Baby - A Journey of Hope and Healing_'. It is a gentle story explaining what is happening to their Mummy. It is a story for them to have the strength to hold on and to guide her towards her healing. It was created with emotion so that a mother can read it to her child and in itself it can be very healing and connective. If she is unable to read it, then the partner or family can read it and offer some respite or answers, but most importantly _hope_ to this beautiful child.

Without adding more layers of guilt or resentment about the situation, it is simply important to be able to be there for them all the time. Give them the comfort, nurturing and love that they would miss, and fill their safety bubble with so much protection and hope. It is hard for them to navigate their way through life without their Mummy and so give them the attention, nurturing and security that they need and deserve.

If friends can arrange play dates, then this is another helpful thing to do to bring more fun into their world. It also gives you a break, which is important too.

Engage with them and allow them the opportunity and the safe space to articulate and share how they are feeling and how this is affecting them. Feeling sad and frustrated is natural, and sharing this with their family is a beautiful life lesson in leaning on those around you for support, when they are feeling lost and confused. They do not have to navigate their way through this alone.

TOOL 7: MINDFULNESS STRATEGIES

It is a stressful and energetically draining experience being present in handling post-natal depression day after day, moment after moment, night after night. I do get it.

It therefore becomes so important to find strategies that best suit you and provide you respite.

Meditation, yoga, journaling and breathing are all effective mindfulness strategies that can help nourish and soothe your nervous system, as well as allowing your mind to calm and be best equipped at facing the stress and strain hour after hour.

Similar to my advice for the Mummy, find your happiness triggers and do little acts of self-charging to keep your spirits high, so that you have the ability to hold on with poise and strength.

It could be some time out just to go to the gym or play tennis. It could be to chat with a friend or go for a run. Find what is an effective outlet for your frustrations, because without channelling them correctly they can fester and explode, which is not beneficial to anyone within the home nor is it allowing you to face the situation with a clear and calm mind.

TOOL 8: EXERCISE

Exercise, whenever and wherever you can! Your mental health is vital and the endorphins that will be released, will flood your system and allow you to handle each day with more clarity of mind, energy and patience.

It is an excellent outlet for your energy and frustration, which can be very therapeutic when you feel stressed and burdened by your reality.

Avoid drinking alcohol in excess, as it acts as a depressant which invariably can make you feel more flat and low if you are continuously leaning on it. Make sure you adhere to the NHMRC guidelines of healthy alcohol consumption, which currently stands at no more than 10 alcoholic drinks per week and no more than 4 on any one day.

Try to eat fresh, *prana* rich (life-force filled) food as much as you can, drink enough water and sleep whenever you can with lots of 'sleep hygiene strategies', that have been listed earlier in this book.

TOOL 9: NO BLAME GAME

As a partner, family or friends, don't enter any blame game about who caused what and try not to deviate from the ultimate task at hand, which is to bring the mother into recovery ASAP.

Everyone needs to offer help and advice filled with love, compassion and kindness. Everyone is human and fallible, meaning that everyone could always do better. There is absolutely no room for blame, anger and frustration at times like this.

Yet, if we work together as a team with the same goal in mind and align for the single pointed focus of healing, then the journey will be smoother together.

As a partner or family/carer, do not make the mother feel worse than she already does by showing your frustrations towards her or the situation. If you do add these layers onto her then more grief, darkness, heavy feelings and the emotions of guilt or shame will breed. It can be so hard to heal the wounds of what is said and done in moments of frustration, *especially* when she is already feeling vulnerable and weak.

Stay and be the anchor that the home needs in this instance, and remember that life is not always easy. Stay committed to being the best partner and support person for her.

TOOL 10: OPEN COMMUNICATION AND ALLOW SPACE FOR HEALING WITHIN YOUR RELATIONSHIP

The truth behind going through a heavy and stressful period like this in a relationship, is that it can create resentment and hostility. In our relationship we have had unhealed wounds or triggers that present at various times, but we allow ourselves to face it eye to eye through open communication, for as long as needed until we have achieved closure.

We could either run away and ignore it, or we could let it fuel into a tumultuous fire that could destroy our future. Yet, we choose at every point, no matter how ugly it may look and feel, to face it, openly communicate and heal those aspects of our being and experience.

I feel that there needs to be forgiveness for your partner and family member for being ill, and for you to know deep in your heart, that she did not do this on purpose or bring pain or hurt knowingly. Biochemistry, underlying nutritive levels and factors outside of her control brought it on and it is vital that your relationship heals all aspects of what presents. I can completely understand how the stress and strain of all of this, can shatter relationships and families.

It would be completely heart breaking to see it happen, but I can empathise with the level of heaviness that enduring an experience like this can bring.

I have included some healing tools that you can work through as a couple, and even as a family member/carer, to help guide and navigate conversations and open communication which I share in the next section. I hope that it can shine some insight and healings into areas that you may need to work on.

During the depths of post-natal depression, I certainly wouldn't recommend hashing out old marital wounds or past family stories. The first and only priority has to be in her recovery. Certainly, if the extent of her depression allows her to articulate and talk through her feelings she may be having, then open communication may allow the air to clear and lighten the tension that may be present, due to not understanding each other. It would be a great idea to go with her to some, if not all appointments at the psychologist or counsellor to work through critical issues together with a trained professional.

Through communication and transparency of emotions, there leaves no room for judgement or misunderstanding. It allows the other person to say unequivocally what they need from you and it allows you the opportunity to rise up and give them what they need.

I feel like when you face something as dark and treacherous as this that open communication, continuously peeling away layers that no longer serve you as a couple, is so valuable.

TOOL 11: SEVEN UNHELPFUL THINGS AS A CARER TO SAY OR DO

These are some insights that I gained as to how best to treat the person who is unwell. I feel that there are things that can hinder progress or build hostility or frustration which later require healing.

Therefore, acknowledging what they are is important to hopefully prevent one from making her feel worse.

1. Never say to 'snap out of it', 'cheer up' or 'it could be worse'. These statements make the person feel like they are choosing to feel that way, and is not placing value on how they are *actually* feeling. Instead, ask them how they are feeling and what you can do to support them. Open questions are less dismissive and critical and most likely to give you an honest response.

2. Do not assume that they will miraculously get better, without any change or action being taken. Without taking steps into the right direction of healing and seeking out help from medical professionals, then it could be a very long road to recovery. Biochemical imbalances do not restore themselves if deeply set-in, and require guidance from a trained professional.

3. Do not stay away from them or avoid them. Even if the situation is frustrating, do not ever take it out on them. Remember, that they are not doing any of this on purpose. Whilst the behaviour may be very taxing, it is not their fault and you must never make them feel worse by what is unfolding.

4. Do not get angry or frustrated with them. If you feel frustrated, then do some exercise, journal it out, speak to a friend and release it in a healthy way. Joining her in counselling can be an effective strategy, to get you both through this stressful period.

5. Do not compare the mother with any other woman or mother, and make her feel worse about herself. No-one

truly knows anyone's actual day-to-day situation. It is not fair to focus on a highlight reel of that person and bring your partner or family member down, especially when she is not feeling herself as it is.

6. Do not talk negatively about your partner in front of any family members, especially your children. It will make your partner feel worse if she hears it and your children may get more confused or detach from her even further, which can make the recovery even longer and more arduous than it needs to be.

7. Do not point out all of the things that she may not be doing and make her feel worse about the whole situation. Help her to complete the tasks or work together in finding the best solution, that would suit the family situation but not highlight anything to make her feel worse. This mother needs to feel held, seen and supported.

HEALTH TIP:

A WATERFALL MEDITATION/VISUALISATION

This is a beautiful meditation or visualisation to energetically clear yourself in the shower. It is a way to cleanse any feelings of stagnation and negativity, as well as re-set your body, mind and spirit to feel refreshed and metaphorically cleansed.

Try it when you are feeling low in mood, your anxiety is heightened or feel like a quick re-set within your system...

+ _Imagine there is a beautiful white light emanating from the sky and is shining directly into your shower faucet._

+ _As the water falls down over your face, feel this beautiful white light cleansing your mind, your thoughts and washing away all of your feelings, that you do not want to harbour within your body any longer._

+ _Allow the water with the warmth of the light to cleanse every cell on your skin and feel it cleanse your body internally, as each drop falls over your entire body._

+ _Imagine this healing light and water wash away all of your worries and stagnant energies down into the drain. Washed away to connect deep into the ocean. Imagine it being able to strip away every morsel and layer of feelings that you want washed away._

+ _Allow it to all dissipate and disappear, away from your body and away from your soul._

+ _Now feel the pure, warm, potent and healing water and light pouring down, to heal your body from the outside in. Allow this to heal your system and feel it as it touches every ounce of your skin, one drop at a time._

+ _Stay in this space and energy for as long as you need it to envelop your entire body. Feel and allow it._

+ _As you finish your shower, wrap yourself in your fresh towel and fully hold your body in this towel and feel the support, nourishment and nurturing that it brings to you._

+ _Hold yourself. Then take this new and enlivened energy with you, as you go about the rest of your day._

CHAPTER 9

HEALING TOOLS

Exercises can be helpful to work through together as partners, in healing and clearing through any unresolved tensions. This by no means replaces the professional services that a psychologist or a couple's counsellor can offer. If you are in any danger or feel like things are very delicate, then I would highly encourage you to both see a health professional as soon as possible, to work through your issues and best equip yourselves in being able to navigate your way through this chapter.

I created these exercises to work through our unresolved aspects as a result of our experience. It was a very connective and clearing process to go through and I felt like we allowed space for honesty and open communication, by partaking in this process.

WHAT TO DO

- Create a calm and serene environment where you both feel comfortable

- Play some relaxing music that you both gravitate towards

- Light a candle or dim the lights, so the bright lights do not activate the nervous system and heighten any anxiety when speaking one's truth

- Set the intention of honest healing and start the process however you feel, is best for you. You may go through the questions that are relevant for you both or you may jumble them up and randomly do them. You may choose to work through them systematically. Rephrase the timing that pertains to your situation, as some may choose to do this in the midst of heightened distress, or perhaps like us, it was after our recovery

There is no right or wrong way to go through this process; however, make sure that you are both energetically and cognitively ready to embark upon this healing. In the throes of the darkness that may not be the best time to broach such topics, unless it allows for clarity to come from it.

Acknowledge your partner and allow space for listening and sharing. Take turns in answering each question to honour both of your needs in the relationship and healing.

It is important to acknowledge that a heavy and delicate situation like post-natal depression *can* have the capacity to create residual or rippling effects, that require nurturing and attention to sift through. By no means can entering the trenches in the thick of a crisis, not result in some trauma or healing that needs to be done; which again I want to be honest in sharing, so that you do not feel alone or isolated in your situation.

Open communication, being raw and authentic in how you are feeling about certain aspects, is what will allow you to be able to shed the trauma and rise into an honest and open relationship, without the heaviness lying on your shoulders and heart.

Take the time to set it down and walk with ease and grace into your future x

EXERCISES:

1. What is it that you want and *need* to heal from this time?

2. What is the best outcome that you want from this healing for our relationship?

3. What is it from *me* that you need to be able to heal this, and to move forward as a couple?

4. What do *you* feel you need to find or heal *within* yourself from this?

5. What is holding you back?

6. What do you feel you are risking by staying held back?

7. What do you have to gain from healing?

8. What action steps can you take right now to begin the healing process and move forward?

9. What action steps can *we* as a couple take right now to begin the healing process?

   Choose an action step as listed below (each step is in detail on the next few pages) or work through the list sequentially if you wish to. You can do this exercise privately and spend as much time as you need, processing and exploring your inner feelings towards it, or do it collectively as a couple;

   - letter writing articulating your feelings
   - anger letter writing about the situation and the people involved
   - forgiveness letter to your partner, yourself and/or others

- cutting the cord of energetic ties
- going back to that time and healing your memories of that time
- meditating on what skills you want to harness to be able to move through this
- a letter to yourself of what you need to let go of

10. Do a symbolic gesture of burning, ripping, cutting the letters to give you a cathartic response and to obtain closure and peace. Fill your heart with loving kindness, compassion and forgiveness to others and yourself. True understanding and appreciation for what this experience brought to you; whether it be good, bad or ugly. Honour the purpose it served you and to give thanks for it, showing up for you and your highest good, should you allow yourself to see it.

11. Write a letter to your future-self telling them what you want that future to look like and ask, what relationship do you want with your partner?

12. What aspects within your relationship do you think work well and what areas can you improve on?

13. What do you feel your *partner* needs more of in the relationship to feel nurtured, honoured, seen, heard and felt in the space of your love and embrace? Ask them and compare, as well as acknowledge what they need and then do the same in reverse.

14. What do you want to see more of and incorporate into your lives, so that you both live the most abundant, wholesome, complete life filled with vitality and pure joy?

15. How do you see keeping up a healthy relationship and healthy communication so this doesn't escalate to such a level again?

16. What are you consciously going to do to live your best self, highest truth and the best version of yourself for your family?

SPECIFIC INSTRUCTIONS ON HEALING EXERCISES

Letter writing articulating your feelings

In a clear and relaxed space, without interruption, pour yourself a glass of wine or a cup of beautiful tea and sit down with an open mind and heart, together with a pen/paper or laptop and be ready to articulate how you are feeling.

Write about what is buried deep within you about the PND, the trauma, the darkness, hardship, how you felt and the feelings associated with the memories. No doubt this will uncover the trauma and reignite the wound, but until feelings are ascribed to it, the emotions will remain dormant within you causing pain and possibly disease vs being able to address it and create a space of healing.

You can write a letter to yourself, your partner or it can simply be a journal type writing to allow you to acknowledge and process exactly *how* you felt during this time.

Anger letter writing about the situation and the people involved

Writing a letter filled with anger towards the situation, directed at a particular person or people, if that is what you feel within your being; will allow that anger, hostility, resentment and fury to come out of your chest, heart and body. It will allow that energy to be poured out onto a real vessel, namely paper.

You do not ever have to give it to that person so there is no reason to be polite, politically correct or to hold back. Rather, unleash as if your life depended on it and you have free rein to let it all flow from your body until you feel lighter, more unburdened and more at ease from the release.

Dealing with emotions, feelings and pent up thoughts can be very exhausting, especially when it brings to the surface things you felt you had parked somewhere for some time. However, keeping it stored within is more likely to leave an imprint of these emotions at a cellular level, and create room for harbouring illness and disease.

It is vital for your best way of living and for those people around you, to help work through the emotions that you are feeling and to acknowledge that this is how you feel. It can only be for your eyes or if you do want to share with your partner, so that they can understand the depths of your position, then you do what is right for you as a couple. Keep in mind that if your partner was the one with PND, that you do not want to trigger any emotions or trauma in them, nor do you want to release more feelings of anxiety and depression. This is not the point of this exercise.

Forgiveness letter to your partner, yourself and/or others

Once you have articulated and worked through all of your deep feelings of anger, frustration, resentment and hostility, it is time to open your hopefully now less-burdened heart, and allow yourself to find forgiveness for all the people referred to in the letter, one at a time.

The feeling and act of forgiveness is one that provides compassion, acceptance and understanding to those people and situations, that have caused so much hurt and pain within you. It is the most important gift that you can give to yourself, even if that person never knows how you felt or that you are forgiving them.

Find the strength to come to a place of pure compassion, acceptance, understanding and forgive them with all of your heart and with every cell in your being.

Whether they did things to intentionally hurt you or not, by carrying the anger within, you are only hurting yourself. In order for you to live a healthy and harmonious life, you need to forgive them for your own inner well-being and peace.

Cutting the cord of energetic ties

Energetically it is important to cut the cord and ties with that person or situation that caused you such grief, as it gives a very good visual representation of that person no longer being attached to your energetic field and sapping your vital life-force.

Imagine this person or situation in your mind's eye with your eyes closed. Imagine they are connected to your belly button with a cord.

Imagine then that you forgive them, thank them for their part in this process and have the internal strength to be able to visually cut the cord tied to you and allow them to float away.

Fill your heart with so much loving kindness and joy, and let that expansion extend throughout your energetic field and shine brightly on all those around you. Where feelings of anger, hostility and resentment are very restrictive, constricted and limited; love, joy, forgiveness and compassion are expansive, and energetically are light.

You will feel so much more freedom from releasing the hold that they have had on you.

Going back to that time and healing your memories of that time

Imagine floating back to that time when all of this trauma was happening, and allow yourself to feel that energy of that space again.

Send loving kindness and healing energy to yourself, partner and everyone that was involved in that time. Allow all of your feelings and memories etched at that time to be filled with healing, unconditional love and so much forgiveness for all that happened. No longer allow that time to have a hold on you, but rather an appreciation for all that it brought you. Allow your heart and mind's eye to be filled with memories of healing only.

Meditating on what skills you want to harness to be able to move through this

Meditation is a beautiful inward tool. It enables us to completely surrender and allow pure internal reflection as to what you need to work through to clear, heal and move on from an experience. This is vital in order to connect and be with your highest self; the unchanging divine light of truth within.

Reflecting on your limited views, mindsets and feelings will allow you to shift and clear what you need to. Ensure that the space is one of non-judgement and pure compassion, in order to live with the growth mindset and releasing the heavy baggage from you, once and for all.

Shedding unnecessary layers that no longer serve you, is the best way to live freely. Reflection is the only way one can do that, unless you are lucky enough for someone to shed awareness on it. Otherwise, you will need to sit and identify or allow it to come to you, as to what you need to transform within yourself.

Just allow and do not force any logic or thoughts. Just sit and allow for any messages to come through, without judgement or resistance.

A letter to yourself of what you need to let go of

The above exercise is more of an inward, internal and reflective process. This exercise would use more of your logical mind and analysis of what you think in a methodical way, of what layers need to shed. It could also be a way to document what came up from your meditation process.

You may find that different things come up based on your logical vs heart space and intuitive mind. Go with it and let in all that needs to come up.

What are you going to do to best support, nourish and honour your partner?

Make a declaration to yourself after your sessions of honesty and sharing with one another, as to what you are going to do to honour your partner and to support and nourish them in the best way possible.

How are you going to show up and meet their needs?

I invite both of you to make a written commitment statement and keep it somewhere where you are both accountable and can refer to it whenever you need a reminder.

CONNECTION HEALING:

In a similar vein to the above healings, you can work through these sequentially or you can mix them up or choose the ones that you resonate with and feel you need the most.

You could work through one exercise once a week or do an intensive one per day. No hard and fast rules! Just go with what you feel is best and have fun in the process!

1. Sit across from each other legs crossed, whilst sitting on a chair, bed or couch...or you may prefer lying down...and give each other a big, huge hug with the timer on for 7 minutes. Do not let go and fully embrace each other for the full duration.

2. Hold each other's hands and look into each other's eyes without talking or looking away for 7 minutes.

3. Each apologise to one another for what you feel you need to after number 2...Declare what you promise to do for the relationship, how you will honour each other and how you will bring yourself into the relationship, to make it the best it can be.

4. Tell the other person 5 things that you love and respect most about them.

5. Ask each other what limiting thoughts, beliefs and traits you want your partner to heal and grow in. Allow space for being honest, without taking offence or being too sensitive. Don't be nasty, but be honest at the same time...whilst being respectful, especially if your partner is still in the throes of her post-natal depression (which is why we worked through these exercises upon my recovery, as I would not have been able to construct any useful contributions).

6. Ask one another what hobby or fun activity you can do together as a couple, and take action to make it happen. It could be painting, cooking or going to a new restaurant once a month.

7. Do a connection challenge, where every day for 30 days, there is one new act of connection...(write a list of things that can be done. You can pull a card each day and it does not need to be only physical in nature! Connection is honouring the other person and could be something like a beautiful shoulder massage). Set a beautiful mood and time aside for real connection and honesty, to heal all the broken wounds inside.

8. The Gottman Institute has an App of card decks to download, that has so many beautiful options to work through if you feel drawn to that.

9. Once you complete the 30-day challenge, then do connection exercises weekly for a few months, then reduce to every two weeks or once a month. It will be very important to keep this up to ensure connection, your needs are being met and true honesty and integrity is being met within the relationship.

This can be particularly helpful and important when children arrive as schedules and priorities change, both feel tired/touched out and energetically zapped. Keeping your connection and honouring your partner is important and can often shine the light on emotional needs that are not being met.

These tools are all things I hope can bring more fun and lightness into your hearts and home. I know first-hand the heaviness that an experience like this can etch onto the minds and hearts of all those affected. Whilst time heals all things, sometimes we all need a helping hand to make the road a little clearer.

I would highly recommend that together as a couple, you do see a counsellor or the psychologist within the triage team allocated to you, so that you can safely navigate through deeper issues with a trained professional. Working through heavy concepts allows for a strong and clear foundation to be set, and how freeing that will feel for both of you. Taking your older children to navigate through their feelings and trauma can be a beautiful thing to do too, as facing our feelings and residual trauma head on will allow everyone to live unapologetically and with *so* much freedom! Who wouldn't want that?!

I hope that by leaving nothing to the imagination as to what I felt like and what I was experiencing, that it can help you connect and find parallels within how you are feeling and to know that help is available outside of these feelings.

I hope that you have gained the courage to move forward and to take the first step.

I hope that you can see through the tools listed, that there are so many beautiful strategies that you can try, one at a time, in order to make your days less painful for you, your baby and your family.

I hope that this has given your heart and soul some much needed solace and hope.

I hope that you have faith, that there *is* so much light at the end of the tunnel...It will come, even sooner than you can imagine...and it will feel even brighter than you remembered x

CHAPTER 10

RESOURCES IN AUSTRALIA

If there is ever a crisis, where the safety of
you or your baby is at risk **CALL 000**

1. LIFELINE:

13 11 14
(Available for crisis support 24/7)
If you ever feel in danger, call them
ASAP

2. BEYOND BLUE:

1300 224 636
(www.beyondblue.org.au)
Resources for mental health
conditions

3. PANDA:

1300 726 306 (panda.org.au)
Perinatal Anxiety and Depression
Australia; specific resources for
pregnancy and the post-natal
period

4. GIDGET FOUNDATION:

1300 851 758
(gidgetfoundation.org.au)

Resources for Perinatal Anxiety and Depression through online resources, Telehealth, Gidget Houses for both mothers and fathers

5. COPE:
Centre of Perinatal Excellence (cope.org.au)

Provide support for the emotional challenges of becoming a parent

6. SUICIDE CALL BACK SERVICE:
1300 659 467 (suicidecallbackservice.org.au)

Nationwide service providing 24/7 phone and online counselling

7. WHOLEISTIC HEALING CO
My Website
wholestichealingco.com

Email address

info@wholeistichealingco.com

Access to other publications/ books, sound healings, products, information, drug information, videos, infant massage resources
Instagram: whole_istichealingco
Facebook: whole_istichealing

8. RELATIONSHIPS AUSTRALIA:
1300 364 277 (relationships.org.au)

Organisation that support respectful relationships across Australia

9. AUSTRALIAN PSYCHOLOGICAL SOCIETY (APS):
1800 333 497
Search functionality for locating psychologists

10. PSYCHIATRISTS	yourhealthinmind.org.au Search functionality for locating psychiatrists
11. HEAD TO HEALTH:	www.headtohealth.gov.au Assists with digital mental health and wellbeing resources
12. KIDS HELPLINE	FROM 5 YEARS TO 25 YEARS 1800 551 800 (kidshelpline.com.au) Free 24/7 call or online counselling services for young people
13. YOUR GP OR OBSTETRICIAN	Can arrange a Mental Health Plan and refer you to psychologists and psychiatrists through Medicare
14. THE GOTTMAN INSTITUTE	www.gottman.com Card decks App to download, also resources to support all family relationships
15. AUSTRALIAN BREASTFEEDING ASSOCIATION	www.breastfeeding.asn.au 1800 686 268
16. PARENTLINE	1300 301 300 (QLD and NT) 1300 130 052 (NSW) Professional phone counselling and support service for parents and carers
17. JEAN HAILES FOR WOMEN'S HEALTH	jeanhailes.org.au National digital gateway for women's health and wellbeing

18. THE MENTAL HEALTH LINE (NSW)

1800 011 511
24/7 operated, staffed by mental health professionals to direct you or a loved one where to go

19. DOMESTIC VIOLENCE

1800 737 732 (1800RESPECT)

20. FAMILY RELATIONSHIP ADVICE LINE

1800 050 321

21. EARLY PARENTING CENTRES IN EACH STATE;

STATE	CENTRE	CONTACT
NSW	KARITANE KARITANE MENTAL HEALTH SERVICE	1300 227 464 (karitane.com.au) 1300 227 464
	TRESILLIAN	1300 272 736 (tresillian.org.au)
ACT	Tresillian Queen Elizabeth 11	1300 272 736
NT AND QLD	ELLEN BARRON CENTRE	(07) 3139 6500
VIC	QEC	(03) 9549 2777
	O'CONNELL FAMILY CENTRE	(03) 8416 7600
WA	NGALA	(08) 9368 9368 (Perth) (ngala.com.au)
	NGALA	1800 111 546 (country)
TAS	WALKER HOUSE- North	1300 064 544
	PARENTING CENTRE- North West	(03) 6477 7323
	PARENTING CENTRE- South	(03) 6166 1605

22. AUSTRALIAN ASSOCIATION OF SOCIAL WORKERS

aasw.asn.au

23. HEALTH DIRECT

healthdirect.gov.au

24. Infant Massage Information   www.babymassage.net.au
    Service (IMIS)   1300 558 608

25. SANE   www.saneforums.org
                                  1800 187 263

26. CARERS AUSTRALIA   1800 242 636

27. MENTAL HEALTH   1300 554 660
    CARERS NSW

28. RAPHAEL SERVICES

(PART OF ST JOHN OF GOD HOSPITALS THROUGHOUT AUSTRALIA,
OFFERING MENTAL HEALTH SERVICES)

29. SLEEP HEALTH FOUNDATION   sleephealthfoundation.org.au

CHAPTER 11

SUMMARY OF ALL TOOLS AS A QUICK REFERENCE GUIDE

<u>SUMMARY OF REFLECTIONS AND TAKE HOME MESSAGES:</u>

1. How we birth does NOT matter

2. We need to be more kind to ourselves, whatever our breastfeeding journey looks like

3. Write a commitment statement to yourself

4. Drop the comparison

5. Research is required into definitive and underlying nutritional imbalances as pre-disposing causes for PND

6. Our identity after having children

7. Confusion of overwhelming information overload

8. Fear of getting in trouble or the implications of speaking out

9. Find your no-fuss friends and tribe

10. PND affects all those around you

11. Body image and self-love of our body after having children

12. Inner self-talk is important to monitor

13. Aspect of control

14. Releasing judgement

15. Releasing guilt and shame by speaking out and receiving help

16. Health is the most important thing and don't be deceived by what things appear on the outside

17. Ayurveda principles as a beautiful way to nourish and support a woman post-birth

18. Importance of the place of infant massage in our healing from PND

19. Need for a connective relationship in pregnancy vs clinical/ masculine approach

20. Dr Shefali's Portal of Pain theory

21. An opportunity to evolve and shift outdated paradigms upon healing to live my best life

22. Need for change and light

23. Listening to your intuition; your inner guidance system

24. Final Word

SUMMARY OF RESTRICTIVE THOUGHTS AND MINDSETS

1. Perfectionist

2. All or nothing

3. Catastrophising, over generalising, jumping to conclusions

4. Negative lens, pessimistic

5. The 'grass is greener' mentality

6. Black and white mentality

7. 'Could have, should have' thinking

8. Control

9. Organised, structured, routine

10. Comparison

11. Masculine mindset vs divine feminine

12. Victim mentality

13. Self-blame

14. Perceiving life as a dress rehearsal vs being present

15. Rigid and needing to study/prepare

16. Fortune telling

17. Fear

SUMMARY OF SELF-HELP STRATEGIES FOR THE MOTHER

1. CBT, IPT, MBCT or Behavioural therapy at a GP or psychologist. Seek medical treatment

2. Manage self-talk and thoughts

3. Working through problem solving

4. Exercise (all exercise, yoga, Ayurvedic yoga)

5. Reduce alcohol to minimal level, if not completely

6. Stay hydrated and reduce caffeine

7. Manage stress (meditation, breathing/Pranayama, a warm bath, grounding activities and scents, access your unique relaxation tool kit of strategies)

8. Reach out to a friend or family member to talk

9. Do something that you normally love to do that sparks you up

10. Turn off the T.V and unnecessary noise or stimulation

11. Support yourself with as much sleep as possible

12. Ayurvedic food, Ayurvedic teas and herbs/spices (Prana rich food, little to no processed and convenience type foods)

13. Ayurvedic practices

14. Infant massage

15. Create an environment conducive to healing

16. Stop worrying about others

17. Be gentle on yourself

18. Gratitude

19. Go out in nature, break up the routine

SUMMARY OF TOOLS FOR THE PARTNER AND CARER/FAMILY

1. Be honest with others as to what is happening and allow help

2. Healthy and Prana/life force rich food is vital during this time

3. Talk to a good friend or support person to vent

4. Take action for your partner

5. Take time off work if possible

6. Nurture your older child that may feel so lost and confused

7. Mindfulness strategies

8. Exercise

9. No blame game

10. Open communication and allow space for healing within your relationship

11. Seven unhelpful things as a carer to say or do

EPILOGUE

This journey of writing and reflecting upon my journey has been deeply healing. The process of going through my learnings, reflections and doing the inner work, has given me a lot of understanding and closure for many aspects within this chapter. Whilst time is the greatest healer of all, this process has allowed for me to navigate through this journey and allowed for deep internal healing within.

My boys shook my world to its *core* on their arrival, in a way we were not prepared for. We as a family reached the depths of despair and darkness, yet we gathered the strength and courage to keep fighting one day at a time, until I was able to return back into my light.

I am so *grateful* for my boys bringing me such an amazing opportunity to step into the person I truly am, and for allowing an awakening of some sort. They have allowed me to fully embrace *all* of life with single pointed presence and connection. My heart has opened more than I thought was humanly possible and they have been my greatest teachers thus far.

Motherhood has allowed me to constantly check-in as to what my triggers are, and then to work through where they came from, what purpose they served and to rise above their hold on me.

I have a new direction and purpose for life, one which I always knew was waiting for me. I have followed my steps one at a time and I have arrived at the place that I am meant to be. That is, to be a vehicle of transparency, so that I can be of service to help other women and their families heal from their journey of post-natal depression.

I will work tirelessly to spread my message and to create practical tools to help *every* woman that requires it. I will work tirelessly to break the stigma and hold that it has on so many cultures and families. I will work tirelessly to advocate for more clinical trials and research into actual measurable underlying causes, to allow for prevention or minimisation for women in generations to come.

I take this opportunity to tell my family; my beautiful boys, brave husband, my amazing parents, my supportive and rock siblings and my 'in-laws' that treated me as their own daughter, just how *grateful* I am for your love, support, holding me and carrying me through my journey, when I had no strength or ability on my own. I love each and every one of you, with every cell in my being and I will forever be *indebted* to you for saving my life twice. I am *so* sorry for causing so much burden and stress during that time and I acknowledge *all* that you did to bring me back to life. My heart is filled with gratitude and things that words may never be able to articulate x

To all of the beautiful women who are reading this and going through the tough road, that may seem unyielding and unrelenting...I *completely* acknowledge where you are and how you must be feeling. I was there. I struggled to keep my faith and resolve with anything. It tested my inner strength, more than anything ever before had.

My message to you is that though it may not feel like it now, you *will* get through this.

I promise.

Hold on, one day at a time.

For your children. For your partner. For yourself.

The beautiful and glorious life filled with light, joy and so much pleasure is waiting for you. The sacred moments that will be available to you, will be in overflow.

You will just need to hold on and take steps towards your healing... The first step being, to speak up to your loved ones and GP/ obstetrician that you recognise the signs within yourself.

You deserve to feel your light and you will. Keep your trust and faith, in whatever it is that gives you solace.

Take one step at a time into meeting your commitment into healing.

Take one action step at a time that resonates with you.

I absolutely believe in you and I know that you will get through this.

Believe in yourself and get ready to feel the bountiful magic of connecting with your children and all of life again. They are patiently waiting for you to come back to them.

Hold on. Be kind to yourself.

Sending you all the strength to get through this.

You've got this beautiful woman x

Instead of writing 'The End', I will finish by saying...

The Beginning (of life, love and a joy like no other) x

GLOSSARY

For some of the abbreviations and Sanskrit words that I have included in the book, this glossary may help to give meaning to some of the words.

WORD	MEANING
Abhyanga	Ayurvedic massage that is done with warm oil. Ideally from a qualified Ayurvedic massage therapist, otherwise *equally* beneficial is self-massage or done at home by a family member to obtain the nourishing benefits after birth.
Agni	Digestive fire that is responsible for the digestion of food and is a crucial aspect of health and well-being within Ayurveda.
Ama	Considered to be un-metabolised waste that is seen as toxic residue, that cannot be cleared or assimilated into the body. It is considered to be the root cause of all disease. It can either be physical residue such as the sticky plaque residue seen as cholesterol in blood vessels or also emotional ama; unprocessed emotions that have not been dealt with or assimilated, that can cause disease also.
Asana	Considered today to be the poses in yoga that are performed, but traditionally in Sanskrit it means the seated posture or position when doing meditation.

Ayurveda	This is the ancient Eastern modality originating in India, that translated from Sanskrit means the 'Science of Life'. Its foundation is that all life forms are made up of the 5 elements of air, space, fire, water and earth. These elements in different combinations form the *doshas* or individual attributes or constitution namely; *Vata, Pitta and Kapha*. Individuals can have one or all three constitution types and this science offers practical tools in nutrition, lifestyle and practices to help balance these *doshas* within your body to maintain an optimum level of health and vitality.
CBT	Cognitive Behavioural Therapy; it is a psychotherapy branch that can be utilised by health professionals and be effective for depression, anxiety, alcohol and drug use, marital problems, eating disorders and severe mental illness.
Dosha	This is the individual energy within the body that can be classified as being *Vata, Pitta or Kapha* based on the combination of the 5 elements namely air, space, fire, water and earth. Everyone has their own inherent and unique combination of *dosha's* that they are born with, which is called ones *Prakruti*. When there is imbalance within the constitution as a result of diet, lifestyle or practices, then it shows with certain symptoms and we call this **Vikruti**.
Guna	This is the Sanskrit word for quality or attribute. We can use this to describe the quality of the mind (*Sattwic, Rajasic or Tamasic*) as well as the characteristics or qualities of each *dosha*.
IPT	Interpersonal Therapy; this is a brief form or branch of psychotherapy that can help in treating anxiety and depression by improving the quality of the clients' relationships and social functioning.

Kapha	This is a type of *dosha* or individual constitution that is made up of the elements of water and earth. General traits of individuals include being loyal, strong, reliable, slow and possibly requiring more energy and motivation.
MBCT	Mindfulness-Based Cognitive Therapy; is a branch or form of psychotherapy that combines a combination of cognitive therapy and mindfulness strategies to form the basis of strategies and overcoming thought patterns.
OB	Obstetrician
PND	Post-natal depression
PNDA	Perinatal Depression and Anxiety
Pitta	This is a type of *dosha* or individual constitution, that is made up of the elements of fire and water. General traits of individuals include being sharp, strong intellect, fiery personality with a lot of determination and drive.
Pragya Aparadha	This is the Sanskrit word for the mistake of our intellect, in causing the loss of 'knowing' or 'remembering' the divine wisdom and the connection to the divine within. It causes choices to be made, that in turn can create more loss of knowingness and this is considered to be one of the root causes of dis-ease.
Prakruti	Inherent constitution or *doshas* of your body that you were born with.
Pranayama	This is one of the Eight Limbs of Yoga that concentrates on the several breathing techniques to control the breath and to unify the body, mind and soul.
PTSD	Post-Traumatic Stress Disorder

Rajasic	This is a Sanskrit word for the mental quality that is active, energetic, passionate, busy, determined, quite 'business-man' like in nature wanting to achieve and acquire more. It is also characterised by the act of action.
Sattwic	This is a Sanskrit word for the mental quality that is pure, clear, full of clarity, peace, equanimity and contentment. It is characterised by an elevated consciousness and having traits of enlightenment.
Savasana	This is a Sanskrit word for the final resting pose that allows for full integration of the Yoga class completed. It allows full connection with the mind, body and spirit to integrate the learnings and connection established during the Yoga.
Tamas	This is a Sanskrit word for the mental quality that is dull, inert, unmotivated and lots of inertia. It is also characterised by the act of completion.
Vata	This is a type of *dosha* or individual constitution that is made up of the elements of air and space. General traits include being erratic, lots of movement, light, cold, active and fast paced.
VBAC	Vaginal Birth After Caesarean
Vikruti	Imbalance of the natural constitution of *dosha's* within the body as a result of diet, lifestyle or practices

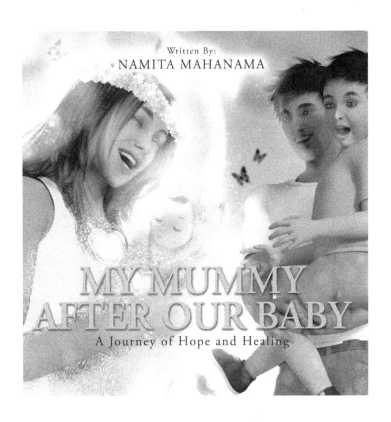

Written By:
NAMITA MAHANAMA

MY MUMMY
AFTER OUR BABY

A Journey of Hope and Healing

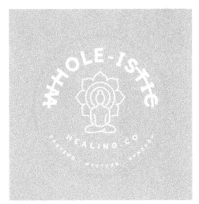

Website: www.wholeistichealingco.com
Email: info@wholeistichealingco.com
Instagram: whole_istichealingco
Facebook: whole_istichealing

ABOUT THE AUTHOR

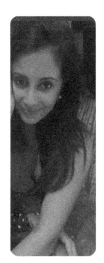

Namita is a mother of two beautiful boys, and became unwell with post-natal depression, from day five until week eleven after giving birth to each of them. She wrote this survival guide resource to help other women and families, by being completely transparent with her experience as well stripping down the condition for everyone to understand what it is, in order to remove the stigma and encourage recognition of the symptoms.

Upon her recovery, she vowed that she would make this journey be filled with more ease and grace, for women moving through it for generations to come. Namita draws upon her first-hand experience, as well as being a pharmacist, studies in Ayurveda, Ayurvedic Yoga teaching and infant massage, to create a myriad of support tools including a children's book titled, _'My Mummy After Our Baby – A Journey Of Hope and Healing'_, to help women navigate through this chapter of life, that she wished she had access to but were not available for her at the time.

Her hope is to inspire, uplift and to encourage all women to speak up to their health provider, in order to allow for their recovery. She also wants to give the message of hope of brighter days ahead.

CPSIA information can be obtained
at www.ICGtesting.com
Printed in the USA
BVHW031249080322
630893BV00006B/97